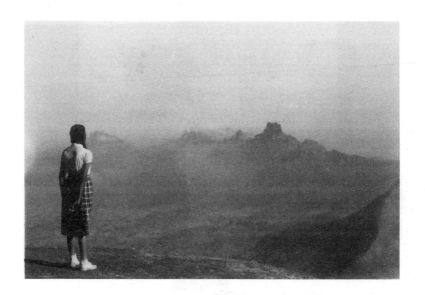

For Mum, who always said,

'I'm not going anywhere. I've still got work to do.'

First published in Great Britain in 2020 by Cassell, an imprint of
Octopus Publishing Group Ltd
Carmelite House
50 Victoria Embankment
London EC4Y 0DZ

www.octopusbooks.co.uk

An Hachette UK Company
www.hachette.co.uk

ISBN 978-1-78840-247-7

A CIP catalogue record for this book is available from the British Library.
Printed and bound in Great Britain

10 9 8 7 6 5 4 3 2 1

Senior commissioning editor: Romilly Morgan
Senior editor: Pauline Bache
Copyeditor: Charlotte Cole
Contributor words: Katherine Ormerod
Art director: Yasia Williams-Leedham
Senior production manager: Katherine Hockley

Frontispiece: Mum aged 16 and just about to leave school.
Back page photograph: Mum just married.

Remember Me?

Discovering
my
mother
as she
lost her
memory

Shobna Gulati

ᴄ

'*Remember Me* is about the complexity of being a mother and daughter and how a child born from political and artistic parents blossoms above all the trauma of migration from India to Britain. I am thankful she has given us a glimpse into her world. Her real world.'

Lemn Sissay

Contents

'I answer the heroic question, "Death, where is thy sting?" with, "It is in my heart and mind and memories."'

Maya Angelou

Introduction: How much do we know ourselves and each other?

This is a story of things that are lost, but also of things that can be found in the most unexpected of places. It is a story of the things you remember and the things you think you have forgotten, the stories we then tell ourselves and what we choose to share with others. It is my story and it is my mother's, and it is about being her daughter. It is about the function of memory within the human construct of time, where we give our daily lives a beginning, a middle and an end. It is also a story about the assumption of shame and the presumption of it too, and of bias and prejudice, based only on the shades of our Brown skins.

We spend our entire lives trying to figure out the rudimentary questions: Who are we when we are with others, and when we are alone? Whose lives have we affected? How did we end up like this? Have we done the right thing? How will we be remembered? These questions entered my mind when I was caring for my mother, and I wondered how she would want to be remembered. I had always believed I had a clear idea of the adult I'd become, and in turn knew who my mother was, both in relation to me and also as a woman in her own right. But the truth is, we never really know ourselves or each other fully. Our memory is an imaginative, creative, destructive and selective place. The memories the brain builds and designs are never quite representative of the life we have lived, and they're not in the stuff we collect and leave behind either. As my mother's memory began to fall apart, I began to see behind the curated memories. And I found a woman who made clear choices grown from a deep, quiet love for her husband and family, and who could live her life fully with fairness and sincerity even when her world fractured.

I never said the words 'I love you' to my mum. Just as she never said those words to me. But we knew.

CHAPTER ONE

Who are we?

I am in a now-empty house, which once belonged to my mum
and dad, which once was the family home, which was my place of
safety with my newborn son, which was my mother's refuge as her
mind began to fail her, and which eventually was the place where
my mother died. I have come back here to sort out her things. I
find myself looking through her old-fashioned green and dark
red photo albums, filled with black card, where, under decorative
delicate paisley tracing paper, I discover images of my sisters
as babies. Their 'first' everything, family outings recorded and
beautifully inscribed underneath with my mother's precise, neat
handwriting noting dates, people and places.

    I see my mum in a black and white photo, with her customary
large circular powder bindi, just like my grandmother's. I imagine

it to be a deep purple, carefully set and perfectly round, in the middle of her forehead between her full eyebrows. She is cheek to cheek with her first-born, in a sari with a matching purple border, captured by her husband, my father, sitting behind the camera with his face pressed up to its glass.

Pictures of my mother and me when I was baby are extremely rare – there are few to be found even of me as a young child. There are plenty of family group shots from India, filled with faces that are familiar but whose names I have forgotten. In these photos I can often be found on my mother's knee, her face set in an apologetic expression, her arms locked protectively around me or pulling my arms away from my face. But as I look through the album, I can't find the individual mother and daughter pictures, the ones that should be there of just us; perhaps those photographs never existed, although I can vaguely remember seeing one. Of course, this is the fate of many a third child: so low down the family ladder that the novelty of first steps and first words are no longer recorded by adulating parents. It wasn't just the two sisters – Hema and Sushma, six and four years my senior respectively – who came before me and dampened my mum's enthusiasm for babyhood mementoes. Nor that there were three of us aged six and under. It was because I was *yet another girl*.

I arrived into the world in the Oldham General Hospital, now known as the Royal Oldham, on 7 August 1966. My mother, Asha, and my father, Dr Kulbhushan Amarnath Gulati, had already established a life here in England. My father had travelled by ship from his home in Matunga, Bombay (which of course became Mumbai in 1995), newly qualified to fill in the skill shortages in the NHS after the Second World War. After a stint in a maternity ward at the Princess Royal Maternity Hospital, on Rottenrow in Glasgow, he had made his way to specialize in paediatrics in Oldham. He was now fully signed up as a medical practitioner on the 'Commonwealth List of The Registrar'. He and other overseas doctors were mostly assigned jobs in the less popular inner-city institutions, and their career progression was often hindered by inherent racist attitudes.

I've often imagined what my dad and mum would have thought of the name 'Rottenrow' – what a place to start your journey in the UK! The name apparently comes from a row of tumbledown cottages infested with rats and goes back to the 14th century or earlier. This Britain, their old 'mother' country, that they had learnt about as Empire's children, the place where streets were paved with gold, had turned into the grim reality of Rottenrow.

When Dad learnt that his wife of seven years had produced another daughter, his response, according to family legend, was 'Oh' and then he hung up the phone (he was working elsewhere in the same hospital). Their third child was supposed to complete the family unit, and, hailing from a North Indian background, it would never be complete without a son. The importance of bearing a son was planted into my mother's head from the moment she married, by her own parents and her in-laws. Thus far, there hadn't been a single grandson for them. Dad's sister had a boy – but that didn't count, because he wasn't 'ours', he wasn't a Gulati. So, my birth wasn't just a disappointment for my parents, it was a setback for the entire family, and it was felt deeply 'back home'.

An airmail letter from her father-in-law, after news of my arrival:

Matunga
Bombay 19
17.08.1966

My dear Asha

You are a brave girl. Is it you who is fond of girls or is it Kulbhushan? I have already named the newcomer – you may call her what you like – Kulbhushan's cousin sisters are Chitra, Reena, Gita, Roopa and Deepa, there is no harm in using the same name as that of one of the cousins. There are hundreds of girls of the same name and with the same surname even. But there is such a rich vocabulary of names. One can always choose a new name or at least a rare name – Hindus have a tendency to name their girls after goddesses and some after gods or after their attendants generally.

We are sure that Hema and Sushma like their sister, if it was a boy, they may have got jealous of him – there is some good in all that God does. We have to submit to His ways and be happy about it.

I can picture this light blue, red-bordered airmail letter, sitting open, by a large brown teapot coddled in a hand-knitted woolly cosy, beside the matching hot mitt my naniji had made. My mother stands by the kitchen sink, deftly rinsing the Fairy Liquid bubbles off the pots with one unsoapy hand, putting them to drain, a misshapen smocked housecoat over a short multicoloured kaftan top and black trousers, all of which conceal her fabulous figure. Her long hair is loosely wrapped around a bun shape at the back of her head. Some orange powder from the bindi on her forehead has fallen onto her nose, tickling it as she swipes the itch with her wet hand, running a yellow stripe down her face in the process. Her husband at work, the older two children already deposited in school. The low murmur of the wireless. On the table the *Daily Telegraph* crossword, already half finished. And baby me, a skinny thing, with a mad crop of black hair, looking up at her fretting.

Rifling through the family photographs, piled high, now in no particular order at the bottom of cupboards, hoarded away for years, the images I can find of me show me in a constant stream of tears – I was a *ro bachche* (a crybaby). Not only was I *not* a boy, I was also a handful. There was always a sense of barely masked disappointment in my mum's face as she tried to hide her embarrassment at the miserable child on her knee. Or I'd be hiding in the back of a picture, where you'd see my head poking out because I didn't want to be in the main photograph. Mum would imitate the sound I made, **'Cheeee cheee chee'**, as I was always whining.

At a certain point, people stop giving you attention for crying all day long, so you've got to find another way to make them notice you. Rather than walk, being the youngest, I was allowed to 'shuffle bottom' (another one of my nicknames), as I made it clear it was my preferred way of travelling about. I came out of the crazy-haired toddler phase, and in photos I appear with a little black bob. Instead of crying, there are 'cheeky-as' grins plastered over my face. I'm smiling as if I've got some mad secret – like I've done the naughtiest thing. Often, I was naughty, very naughty. I modelled myself on Snoopy, wearing two pigtails to imitate his ears, and, as he wasn't a person, I felt a kinship with him because I'd always been marked out as different growing up. I was also trying to love my growing nose, so I told myself I looked like him and I was cool like him too. But really I was Linus.

I had no choice but to fill the space left for me. I spent most of my childhood trying to please my parents and trying to be everything for them. Craving validation and getting attention shaped me for decades. I'd always be desperate to entertain and be what others wanted me to be, even when there was little to no chance of success. I became used to trying regardless, especially for my mum.

The role you adopt and play among your parents and siblings is almost impossible to escape. Hema became the one who had to fight for everything and babysit the rest of us, and she was made to feel her responsibility. Sushma cleaned up after all of us and kept order and the peace. She was the family's mediator – everything had to be shared equitably. And I was the squeaky wheel in the well-oiled unit, the 'pipsqueak'.

I made myself constantly available to my father and became a tomboy who watched football and cricket with him. I kicked stones waiting for him to come out of the members-only all-male clubhouse at Old Trafford cricket ground, and held his hand as we walked into the football ground to watch Manchester United. I was about as high as the bum cracks of the other supporters, tripping over their flared trousers. We went with a packed lunch and red flask of tea, made by me, supervised by Mum. I was in charge of the food and drink and the very important ticket wallets. Dad talked players, managers, the offside rule and tactics and I sagely nodded along.

Then, the minute I was with my mum, I turned myself back into a pretty little girl, wearing her homemade dresses, being interested in what she was cooking and what was on the wireless or at the theatre, or talking about dance. I played both parts well and with equal measure as and when they were required, because by doing so I would prove I was special after all.

Mum was raised in a formal, traditional household, with a lack of tactility that she passed on to her own daughters. There were no big hugs, no obvious demonstrations of love or affection from her. There was a part of her that was unknowable, or at least detached – as though you could never quite reach her. I was extremely wary of her, not just because she was so insular, but also because she was strict as hell. She made clear the standards she expected and woe betide you if you didn't live up to them. But this was exactly how she had been brought up; she was following rules that had been stringently ingrained into her.

Discipline was wielded by the *chappal* (a type of leather sandal) or a hand, accompanied by our mother swearing in Hindi or Punjabi. Often I was naughty, very naughty, and I'd get called *sewer ki dum*, a pig's tail, or *ullu di patthi*, the daughter of an owl (because owls are stupid in Indian culture, despite what the Ancient Greeks say). I was always *gadha*, a donkey. Donkey was Mum's favourite, but pig's daughter and owl's child also featured heavily. **'What have I done to deserve this? Hai Rabba!'** (Oh God!) was also a familiar curse from my mum. When I discovered what the words actually meant I'd reply, 'Well then, you must be an owl, a pig and a donkey if I'm the daughter.' A quick backhand slap would be her response.

But it was Dad who did most of the smacking. Mum gave you a backhander if you were near, but it was my dad who chased me down. The bathroom door in Mum's now-empty house still has no lock on it, as it was repeatedly broken by Dad in his pursuit, although by the time he'd arrived at my favourite hiding place (between the toilet and the bath) his anger had dissipated, and he couldn't reach into this tiny gap anyway. I always fought back and would say this or that wasn't fair. Disagreeing with your parents in our culture means the same as disrespecting them. There is no nuance, no grey area. But I was constantly disagreeing and questioning everything.

For example, at Diwali, we would go to the temple for readings of the ancient Sanskrit epic of the Ramayana, and hear the story about the exile of Ram, his wife Sita and brother Lakshmana into the forest for 14 years. Sita is abducted by Ravana, the ten-headed demon king, and then rescued by Ram and an army of monkeys. But before she is restored to her husband, in order to prove her chastity, she has to enter the fire.

'Why did Sita have to walk through fire when she was the one abducted by the ten-headed demon king? She wouldn't have gone near a demon with a barge pole, let alone one with ten heads... Why on earth did Ram have to test whether she was pure or not? There's no way she'd have kissed him. She had been kidnapped against her will!' And, of course: 'Why do I have to do chores all the time? It's like child labour...did you just have children so we could be put to work?' I was always one for drama and extremes.

I think my parents enjoyed it to an extent, but they also worried about this questioning, which was, in their eyes, so controversial. In fact, one of my other names was 'Little Miss Controversy'. I'd pick fights, I'd say things without any filter, I would not be compliant. I'd say 'NO!' They worried I wouldn't become a doctor, lawyer or engineer...

That I'd be the one who'd disgrace the family.

I can remember the day when everything changed.

In early November 1970 a little brother arrived. I'd just turned four and I had no clear comprehension that he was coming beforehand. My parents named him Rajesh, which means 'ruler' or 'god of kings'; he was their miracle child. It was the luck of the draw that I was the third daughter while he got to be the first grandson.

My mother had a bout of German measles when she was pregnant with him, so there was a lot of anxiety around the birth. There was even talk from medical professionals of the potential need to perform a termination, but my mum was having none of it. It was her utter determination and resistance to the pressure from doctors that led to her baby prince arriving safely.

Sadly, Dadaji (my paternal grandfather) had died the year before, back in Mumbai, and would never know the joy of the grandson he had been yearning for. My dadiji (grandmother) adored her new grandson. She met him on a quick trip we took to India during his early years – Mum and Dad wanted to show him off to her and the rest of the family. That was the visit when Raj also had his first haircut, in a traditional Hindu ceremony known as a *mundan*. There are some lovely photographs of Raj sporting a new shorter haircut, though Mum couldn't bear to shave off his gorgeous curls because it would make him less beautiful.

That reticence was in stark contrast to how she had treated me one summer when, much to her horror, my hair had become knotted and tangled as I played wild in the dirt with the cats on a farm holiday. In response she cut off all my hair into a severe boy's crop, without a second's thought – so at four I had shorter hair than my brother. It wasn't the best look, but it grew out into the bob and my newest nickname became 'Palm Tree', because she tied up my fringe with a bobble.

Photographs from India show Raj wearing a beautiful white silk traditional *churidar pajama* and a deep maroon embroidered waistcoat, kissing our bedridden grandmother on her cheek, her smile so, so wide, as she beamed with pride. Actually, in the years that followed my brother's birth, my dad's younger brothers got married and had two sons each. My dadaji and dadiji would have been so thrilled.

The photo albums are full of pictures of Mum and Raj. Certainly, no shortage there. Photographs in full 1970s technicolour. And Mum is even *kissing* him in them. He is the podgiest, cutest baby boy, with milk chocolate brown button eyes, a mass of loose curls and the most adorable smile, in direct contrast to photos of me as a baby – skinny, displeased, with a bottle in my mouth.

I became even more difficult, especially about him, causing more trouble with my moods and crying, developing a deeper and deeper attachment to a comfort blanket I had named 'shawli'. Soon after Raj was born, a new dynamic between us kids formed, and it became a divide between the older two and the younger two. Even though Raj was four years younger than me, much to my chagrin I was coupled with him. It definitely contributed to my immature behaviour and I remained very childlike for a long time. Any attention, even if it was a reprimand to my misbehaviour, was better than no attention at all.

We children were brought up by parents who themselves were children of the Empire. My mother was born in England in 1940, because my grandad, Jamna Das, was working on the British railway network as an electrical engineer, and my grandmother, Shanta Malhotra, had come with him. They learnt a lot from his time living in the north of England – around Crewe, Bolton and Southport, where Mum was born. My granddad was often chased down the street by young boys in shorts on bicycles shouting, 'Hey Indian! Where's your bow and arrow?' My grandparents lodged with a landlady, whose 18-year-old daughter would sit in the tin bath in the front room and shout to my grandad to come and scrub her back, much to my grandparents' horror. My mum always delighted in telling us how she was the only baby in the

Christiana Hartley Maternity Hospital in Southport to have hair on her head. Her British beginnings were certainly a part of her identity, something which her parents encouraged, despite the racism they faced.

When Mum was about one year old, they travelled 'back on the boat', a seemingly endless, precarious journey home, avoiding the U-boats. Our mother regaled us with the story of their long ocean-liner journey from England, a chronicle passed down to her by her mother. Liverpool to Mumbai, going around the Cape of Good Hope and stopping in Durban, as the Suez Canal had closed due to the war and they needed to refuel. The magnificence of their big ship among all the smaller boats around the Southern Tip of Africa. The journey took months, the adults occupying their time by looking after baby Asha, reading books and playing bridge and deck games with a handful of other young Indians leaving their memories of Blighty behind.

It was in Durban that they experienced another kind of racism. It was an overt, full-on, less sophisticated attack, which felt markedly different from the way they had been treated in either Colonial India or England. My grandfather had visited the cinema to watch a film with his friends, and as the lights came on in the interval they were rudely challenged by the ushers as they were apparently sitting in the wrong section...Unaware of the laws of segregation in pre-apartheid South Africa, they had taken the seats they had been given. My grandfather was very fair skinned with dark green eyes, and he was dressed in dapper western clothes, so his 'colour' and attire must have confused the ticket office who sold my grandparents tickets for the 'whites only' section.

As legend has it, my grandfather stood up to the ushers and they continued to watch the second half of the film, albeit stung by the visceral racism they had encountered. They had bought their

tickets and they were damned if they were going to forgo getting
what they had paid for. What had shocked them the most was
that Durban on the surface seemed so multi-ethnic, such a mix
of people and cultures – more so than either England or India.
To experience such undisguised, public prejudice was something
they would never forget.

After returning to Mumbai, my grandfather became one of
the first superintendents of the Indian Railways after the British
left – one of the first Brown people with a leading role in his field.
Even though the railways were built on the blood, sweat, taxes and
tears of the Indians, all you hear in Britain is 'we gave the railway
to India'. But the truth is that they were built because of the
aggressive way the British ruled India, and built off the minds and
bodies of those they colonized. My grandad was very much one of
those minds and bodies.

As the first-born daughter, Mum didn't grow up with quite
the same level of familial disappointment as I did, but with three
brothers arriving afterwards in quick succession she certainly
knew her place as a woman. Her father was very traditional about
women's roles and she wasn't encouraged to to follow the full
gamut of academia. Her father's words rang in her ears: 'Boys don't
make passes at girls who wear glasses'. He believed no one would
marry her if she was too intelligent, and so he prevented her from
wearing spectacles even though she was extremely short-sighted.
As a young woman, Mum was naive, docile and deferential,
exactly as she was supposed to be, but this would only be in the
beginning of her story.

The elder two of Mum's younger brothers were sent off to
boarding school, and my mother and her baby brother, the apple
of their mum's eye, stayed at home with their parents as they were
posted to different places around the state of Maharashtra. Her

fondest memories were of the Railway Colony in Tharkurli, a big old colonial bungalow which stood on a small hill. Inside it had vast rooms, four-poster day beds, beautiful Victorian and Indian wooden furniture bedecked in ancient fabrics, and modern Indian art, religious figurines, and bookcases overflowing with books and old issues of *Reader's Digest*s. The side of the house had a long veranda which looked over the beautiful gardens of lotus flowers, rose, hibiscus and jasmine, where her parents took tea and namkeen (a salty snack), played bridge or had a long, cool whisky and water as a 'sundowner'.

Mum proudly told us that she travelled alone on the train to school in Mumbai and that the manservant, Manohar, met her at the station to walk back home. She bought treats using her saved pocket money of 4 anas and 25 paise to buy Rowntree's Fruit Gums or salty potato crisps or, her absolute favourite, peanut chikki (brittle) bought from a coffee shop called Friends. She also recalled, even more excitedly, a proper cup of tea that she had in a proper china cup in Brandon's (the dining area of the restaurant at the Victoria terminus railway station, originally meant solely for the officers of the British Raj). If she missed the 16.20 train after school, she could have sandwiches on her dad's account while she waited for the next train.

After a stint at the prestigious Elphinstone College, her parents enrolled her into the College of Home Science at Nirmala Niketan in Mumbai to learn how to manage a household in preparation for marriage. Mum used to joke with us that she went to 'finishing school'. At the time, Dad's friends teased him saying she wouldn't be a brilliant home-style cook and would have too many fancy western ways. They said all he would get was cucumber sandwiches. She was enrolled in the diploma course in Home Science for two years. Subjects included physics, moral science, hygiene, sewing, child psychology, mother craft, first aid/home nursing, textile and laundry theory, nutrition, interior decoration and household management.

The ethos of the college left an indelible mark on my mother. I found a college magazine in one of the drawers at Mum's. The director's message:

> **You have come here to prepare yourself for life, to learn how to be efficient home-makers and good wives and mothers. The average person might think that this is a sixth sense for women, but you know that training is necessary so that you can maintain the high standards you have set for yourselves.**
>
> **Your presence in this Institute means that you have already understood that every woman is called by God to be the shining light of her home. If she is to be the pillar of strength and happiness on whom each member of the family will instinctively lean for comfort and guidance, she must learn to give herself unselfishly, with intense love. This is the idea that we wish our motto to convey to you: The highest law of love is service. Every moment of your daily life in your home will be one of service to others and it should be a service of love. Through all that you are taught in this course you are unconsciously imbibing this ideal.**

The rest of the address goes on to cover how important a woman's role is in social welfare and how, by the end of the course, she would be ready to serve because she would have had the opportunity of acquiring the fundamentals of social work in college.

This was the blueprint of how Mum lived as a married woman. The journey of life that she embarked on, her spark of determination and that light that she knew she had, had all been instilled into her psyche, 'unconsciously imbibing this ideal', through her formative years at the college. Nearly all her actions have their basis in the school's motto. She was also the product of parents full of pedantry and traditional values; she was the oldest sibling and a *girl*. She was never going to sacrifice the respect she deserved from her brothers, or from anyone else for that matter. And she brought this attitude to everything she did. This part of her education trained her mind, and consequently all our lives, in ways that she probably couldn't have imagined when studying laundry theory. Who knew that how to wash your clothes could have such a formative effect on a young woman's mind?

My parents' marriage was arranged between their families, who had known each other for decades. When my mum's parents lived in Matunga they moved into a building called Chaya on College Road, living on the first floor, and they made friends with the Gulatis in Adenwallah Road, Africa House. After Partition, Matunga was home to many groups of Punjabi families. Mum often said she hung around with Dad's younger brothers and she'd see him and think how handsome he was. Actually, they grew up to both be very good-looking – she particularly so, a goddess straight out of Greek mythology, with long, long legs and broad shoulders, a proper bosom and tiny waist.

And so, on 18 November 1959, my parents married. Since that day, my mother always wrote her name with a smile and flourish: Mrs Asha Gulati. She was so proudly in love with the man with whom she now shared a name.

In order to become Mrs Gulati, Mum had to agree not to

eat aubergines, indeed she was prohibited from it by her in-laws. Apparently one of the Gulati ancestors had been saved by the aubergine plant and, out of respect, every married woman who held the surname would have to honour aubergines by not eating them. Before her marriage, they had been one of her favourite vegetables, and although she would dutifully cook them for us children, she never ate them herself.

My mother made other sacrifices for my father too. For instance, every Monday was Mum's fast for the continued health of my dad. It was like a form of penance, but I could never work out if it was cultural, religious or indeed just a Punjabi thing. (One thing I am sure of is that it definitely was a patriarchal thing.) She would prepare all our food for us throughout the day but only allow herself one bowl of milk and Shredded Wheat, or a meal with no added salt or sugar, so simple it was without flavour. I would admire her but also feel slightly frustrated; my dad didn't do anything like that for her and I would tease him that he never fasted for her health. I recall him doing it once to show his appreciation and we all found it hysterical because he was so bad-tempered that day.

Ten months later, straight out of medical college, my father left his heavily pregnant wife to study child health in the UK. He was to take advantage of training within the National Health Service in the hope he would become a paediatrician. A couple of days after he left, Hema was born, in early September 1960. Dad received the news by telegram while he was at sea. All their community 'aunties and uncles' (absolutely everyone is an aunty or uncle, blood relation or not, regardless of where they are in the familial line) were secretly counting on their fingers the timeframe of baby Hema's arrival, making sure all was in order and they had indeed adhered to the rules of 'no sex before marriage'. The story goes that Aunty Karnakaran had given Mum orange juice and caster oil to speed up the onset of labour – Mum's face creased up into a grimace when she recalled that moment.

Dad arrived in Marseille on a ship called the *Viet Nam*, then travelled to London and shared in the welcome hospitality of 'relations': my mum's father's brother's son's home in Hertfordshire. 'Uncle Bill' (as we affectionately called him for short, although his real name was Harbans Lal) had already settled in England, and married 'Aunty Stella' before Partition. Aunty Stella was 'Anglo-Indian', a loaded term used at the time of the British Raj for people with mixed ancestry. Mum's descriptions of Aunty Stella were slightly jaded, as she'd had to live with her when she first arrived in England too. Mum would tell us of Aunty Stella saying my dad had borrowed eight pounds off them so he could travel to his first job in Scotland and had never paid them back. She could never let this go, even though Dad arrived in England with a whole five pounds in his pocket.

On arrival in Glasgow Dad found there was no record of him going into further training, so he was called into work immediately and began a stint at the Maternity Hospital on Rottenrow. Much like today, in the midst of Covid-19, many young doctors had to step up to the plate before they were fully qualified. The newly formed NHS desperately needed doctors and, led by the call of the then Minister for Health, Enoch Powell (who, ironicially, would later deliver the infamous 'Rivers of blood' anti-immigration speech), my father and other Commonwealth citizens moved to Britain under the ruse of 'further training', when they actually just desperately needed the staff.

In Indian culture, it's expected that a son's wife joins her new in-laws' household immediately after the marriage. So for nearly a year Mum stayed with my grandparents, living the typical daughter-in-law life. Her mother-in-law was confined to bed even back then, and they needed another woman in the house to help. Her role was the older sister-in-law, the *bhabi*, and she was expected to manage the domestic situation. Her younger sister-in-law also lived there. Mum couldn't bear the thought of two years away from her husband, but her in-laws demanded she follow tradition.

However, it just so happened that one of her father's friends, who was a travel agent, had come to the house for a visit with her in-laws, and it somehow came up that Mum was born in England. The travel agent mentioned how easy it would be to obtain a British passport if Mum could prove her country of birth. Despite her apparent meekness, Mum's steel came to the fore. She realized that the proof of her birth would be on her mother's passport, and within ten days of that meeting she had rustled up her own new British passport from the British consulate. With financial support from her own father, much to her new father-in-law's vexation, by February 1961 she had boarded the next Boeing 707, tiny baby in tow, with a one-way ticket to Oldham, via Aunty Stella.

My father was there to meet her and their child. He was wearing his blue suit – he had one brown one and one blue one, made for his wedding, and Aunty Stella had told him to wear the blue one, because 'Indian men look better in blue'. (In true old Empire style, Aunty Stella's comment reflected the inherent colourism endemic in society, something that she probably also had to face, that my dad's darker skin would be complemented by blue.) My mum was just delighted to be reunited with my father at last, whatever he was wearing. They could finally embark on their married journey together. My parents' story is a genuine love story.

When Mum first arrived up north, her immediate environment wasn't at all what she was familiar with. Doctors lived in the hospital where they worked or in digs close by. Although there were a few other 'Indian' doctors there, they were mostly single: no children, no wives. Mum, Dad and baby Hema lived in all sorts of accommodation: including in Swinton at the Royal Manchester Children's Hospital, and in Pendlebury at 178 Manchester Road, where Mrs Quinn, the landlady, often checked that the flat was kept clean by its new 'foreign' tenants, exclaiming that 'she'd never seen the bath so clean'. (Mum and Dad didn't go in for long soaks. They would have a 'bucket bath', which was a bucket filled with a mixture of boiling and cold water that you poured over yourself, sitting in an empty bathtub, with a little bowl called a *lauta*. It stems from a tradition they had brought with them, of always saving and conserving water.)

Dad took the responsibility of providing for his first-born very seriously and would be on duty all the time as a junior doctor to fulfil that obligation. Mum would wait up for him, preparing only very basic meals. They never really drank coffee or much tea.

Sushma was conceived above a dental surgery, which was often joked about as she eventually became a dentist. My mother often said, **'Fate, Shobna, isn't it? Things have a funny way of turning out.'** After the birth, my mother's mother had sent her some small gold earrings with a clear white crystal to celebrate, alongside a cutting from a newspaper from 'London' (that's how the whole of England was referred to back in India). The headline reported on an escaped criminal and it contained a note from my grandmother asking Mum to be careful when wearing the earrings if she was going out in case she ran into this man.

So, there my mum was, with one lively toddler and one curly-haired babe-in-arms, catching the bus on her own, trying to navigate her way around and find a way to do the shopping within budget. I often imagine her at 23, carrying the bags and my sisters, all alone, so far from home, weighed down with responsibility. It was in 1962 that Dad was diagnosed with late-onset diabetes and my mum was quietly blamed for it in another missive from her father-in-law, who said that Dad had 'got the rich man's disease'.

But their newest flat, in the hospital, was very lively and it became central to the hospital's social scene. Two other doctors – Dr Issac, often clutching a tin of fish, and Dr Agarwwal – came around to play cards during on-call stints, and Mum would cook food for them. The flat became known as Joe's café – Joe being a nickname of Dad's given to him in Scotland because they thought he looked like the pianist and singer Joe Henderson.

My mother loved learning about all the hospital's 'goings-on', as she called them, as sometimes illicit relationships formed within a very tightknit community of overseas doctors and nurses. It never occurred to her that her husband would be unfaithful, but plenty of people tried to falsely implicate him with this or that nurse. He was very popular and handsome. 'Do you trust your husband with Phylis? She has been dating another overseas Muslim doctor.' The inference being that Phylis was the type of woman who fancied all Indian doctors. Microaggressions of racism and sexism were rife in the small community. Mum's eyes were being opened for the first time.

My family moved to a small house on Abbey Hills Road in Oldham just before I was born. It was a little terrace with a lean-to toilet outside. My granny always used to laugh at it and say she couldn't believe that her daughter was choosing to live in a home with an outhouse – after all, the family had indoor upright 'western' toilets in India at the time, not even a squat latrine. This was my first home, but we eventually moved into the hospital because it had central heating, instead of the small wood fire in the living room in Abbey Hills. The temperature of their home was incredibly important to Mum and Dad: the north was so cold.

Then it was decided to go back to India. With three daughters under six, it would be easier for Mum to manage with support and help from relatives. Dad would drop us off in India, then wind up things in England and come back home. But it didn't quite work out. Hema and Sushma's Hindi-speaking school literally blew away – it had just been a tent. My mum couldn't stand being away from Dad again, especially under the jurisdiction of her parents and her in-laws, who thought that everybody had become too Anglicized. (As if to underline this point, Sushma would often whisper into Mum's ear, 'Do they have a toilet like Oldham?' You see, the toilet at our paternal grandparents' Africa House in Matunga, Mumbai, was 'a hole in the ground'. As children, we were all so afraid of falling in, because our little feet would never fit the anti-slip foot markers on either side. Plus, to my complete horror, as I squatted I could see the antennae of what I imagined to be a large cockroach in the corner of the bathroom. Every year we visited as children it was there, waiting. Then just like that, in my late teens, the whole place was refurbished and the cockroach was gone.)

By the end of May 1967, good fortune befell the family as my father became a GP, with a salary upgrade and the ability to buy his first family home, 21 St Albans Avenue, a detached house (with indoor bathroom and central heating) in Ashton-under-Lyne, for the princely sum of £4,500. My mother was quickly back on a plane to England.

Soon after the move to St Albans Avenue, Mum received a letter from one of her old school friends, Vatsala, who remained in India, married with two children:

Your mum had written that you have shifted into your own house, are you going to settle in England for good? I presume Hema and Sushma are schooling. Does Shobna trouble you a lot? Do you have any domestic help?

Asha, do you remember our college days? It's strange how quickly time flies and after a couple of years we will be old fogies!

Are the English well disposed towards Indians?

It's strange to think those girls, who in themselves were so similarly brought up, started their married lives so differently and worlds apart (and nice to see that my reputation preceded me too!).

This time, irrespective of 'how well disposed the English were towards them', Mum and Dad were to settle here for good.

All this movement between India and England meant there was a constant cultural dance at home with the accented consonants of Lancashire English...

The *dhas* and *khas*,

the *a ahs* and the *i ieees* of Hindi

In the mix of that was my dad's shouts of 'Hem, Sush, Sho. Hem, Sush, Sho.' He'd say it endlessly, usually to get him some cheese and biscuits (why else would you have daughters?). More often than not it was me who came, of course.

We existed in a sea of swirling bilingual conversation. My parents spoke to each other in Hinglish, a combination of Hindi and English, even though they were both Punjabi, because Mum thought that the Punjabi language sounded too coarse. I had lessons in Hindi as a young teenager, but it was never a focus, because English was always what Dad wanted us to speak.

This was all part of his big cultural assimilation project – he brought us up very much to fit in, at least outside the home. He didn't mind when people called him Joe instead of his own name, Kulbhushan. He liked it. He even would refer to himself, on occasion, as Joseph. He bid us do everything we could to be British. His philosophy was: at home, we can be different, wear cultural clothes, do cultural things, speak a different language and eat different food, but out *there* we speak English, we wear western clothes and we can eat beef if we want to (despite being born Hindus).

We never took time off for religious holidays. If it was a big religious festival like Diwali, the Festival of Lights, we got together as a family to light candles, sing the *aarti* and do a short prayer or *puja*, and Dad and Mum would go out dressed up to the nines to friends' parties that involved a lot of eating, drinking and card games. It is customary on Diwali night to gamble – Goddess Lakshmi would be impressed and ensure her goodwill for abundance. But this was our 'secret' cultural life, in our home and among some friends; around everyone else we kept to their rules. Oldham was Rome and we were to do as the Romans did.

Another aspect of this assimilation (and continuing the values that Mum was taught at Nirmila Niketan), saw both Mum and Dad heavily involved in charitable organizations and volunteer work. Mum was thrice president of the Inner Wheel of Crompton and Royton District 128, the group for wives of the local Rotarians (in 1979, both she and Dad were president of the Inner Wheel and the Rotary Club respectively). When Raj and I were young, we would accompany them to conferences in different parts of the country, take part in fundraising and spend time with the vulnerable in organized trips to the seaside and tea dances.

Finally there was our education. My dad's family was very different from my mum's, although they were both Punjabi. The importance of the education of girls stemmed from my dadaji, despite his views on the 'value' of boys. After Partition he made sure that his own little sister, who ended up living with him and his wife alongside all his female children, was educated to a good academic standard – my Great-Aunty Channo became a very well-respected teacher who never married. (Another Gulati, who perhaps didn't follow a traditional route.) My eyes always lit up when Mum spoke of her as the one who hadn't followed a well-trodden path. My dad's sisters had been educated and one of them became a world-renowned doctor who set up a women's health hospital in Agra, which still exists as a centre of excellence in IVF today. But when it came for Hema to go up to secondary school, the local Catholic school wouldn't take her, as it did not take other religious groups, so we upped sticks and moved into Oldham proper, where we all went to the private grammar school. Even though Dad was a dyed-in-the-wool socialist, it felt to him that it was the only place where our differences might count in our favour, rather than against us. He had no other choice.

I didn't feel different inside, but no matter what we did, living in Oldham in the 1970s, I was never going to escape how the people around me saw and reacted to my difference. With my skin the colour it was, I was never going to fit in. Even my junior school teacher would point out my difference in a roundabout fashion, saying, 'Shobna Gulati, you think you're the bee's knees,' when I was no more naughty than anyone else. My eight-year-old self would look at her in wonderment, trying to figure out if bees actually had knees.

Even though I didn't think my skin colour was a consideration, everyone else did. That is, everyone else on the outside. The irony

was that, although we did everything we could to strip ourselves
of our religion and heritage when we were outside the house, the
outside only judged us on the way we looked and the colour of
our skin. I'd be called a Paki, a Nig Nog, a Wog or the 'N' word. I
couldn't really work out why they thought I was so different, so
I'd often come back with cuts and bruises or a knocked-out tooth
from fighting. My father always told me to not get involved in any
fights. If he found out through local gossip – I certainly didn't tell
him directly – he would say, 'You can't ever win, Shobna.' There
was also a presumption, by the outside, that I grew up in some
kind of spice shop, with secret recipes and 'authentic' Indian food.
Did I heck! This misconception has followed me through my life
and career. No matter what the job, the opening first-day gambit
in a bid to get to know me is, invariably, 'Ooo I love curry, do you
make it?' or else, 'I made this wonderful curry last night, I do love
spicy food' (as if I actually care). The imprints of Mum's shopping
lists neatly written in little notebooks, frugally kept through the
decades because they still contained spare pages at the back, tell
of meals made from:

milk
bread
eggs
butter
potatoes
sugar
Weetabix
tinned fruit

There were no spices on these early itemized lists, apart from salt
or pepper. Of course, this was also because a lot of that wasn't

easily available back then. You couldn't get your daals in neat little packets from the supermarket. In Oldham, Rice Krispies became a substitute in bhel and chaat mixes, with a combination of tomato sauce for sweetness, PLJ (lemon juice) for tang and HP, that Great British sauce, to add that semi-authentic flavour of tamarind, the irony of the British Raj and their cultural appropriation, smacking us in the face at teatime. Just after school we might have a spicy salty snack (namkeen), or just a bag of Golden Wonder cheese and onion crisps and a hot cup of tea. Spicy scrambled eggs, undey ki bhurjee or bhujia, were served on buttered hot toasted double-roti (my mum's nickname for white sliced bread). It was the 1970s, the era of the pineapple upside-down cake – this was about as exotic as ingredients got in the supermarkets at that time.

After all, my mother had studied food at Nirmala Niketan, where she had been taught to cook western-style food. Indian food as we know it hadn't found its footing in Britain yet, and certainly not in the north. 'Curry houses' were at a minimum and you would only find them around manufacturing mills and the textile industry, in places like Bradford and in the wholesale and textile district of Manchester, now gentrified and called the Northern Quarter. For the Indian doctors who came over to the hospitals, those special cafés or *dhabas* and those community food shops were not to be found, because there just wasn't a big enough community there, at that time. Many doctors had also married 'English girls', the adjective used to describe anyone white who was not from 'back home' and so they too ate English food. Nobody at that time, Mum said, would go out for an Indian meal.

Letters from India, from Mum's in-laws and parents, contained recipes and tips on how to flavour food. My dadaji drew on his experiences of eating in England back in the 1940s. But we did have some traditional Punjabi cooking. I can remember suitcases full of food, snacks and spices coming over when any family or friends came from India and the enormous sacks of chapati flour and rice which would arrive from a wholesaler somewhere in the UK. Sometimes there was a little bulge at the bottom and to our complete horror you'd find a dead mouse. The sacks lived in the garage, and it was my job to sort the contents out. I had to clean the rice and daal by spreading it out onto a huge stainless steel thali and picking out the stones and the rice husks.

When it came to the chores Mum was at her matriarchal best. We all had to do jobs and it felt like they ruled your entire day. Not much sitting down for a Gulati girl. The only way to actually do well in our household as a girl was to polish the taps until they shone, help Mum clean all the daals and the rices, and keep your hair tidy. (I did my best, but usually fell short and got a backhand for my transgressions – usually something to do with my quick wit and answering back. I didn't mean it to be me who was always provoking, but somebody had to ask the difficult questions, even though it was disrespectful to challenge your elders.) We took it in turns to prepare the kitchen for dinner, work with Mum to make the dinner, be the serving girl or clear the kitchen after dinner – just us girls, of course. I was good at the prep and watching Mum's methodical cooking, being on hand in the kitchen as Mum's sous-chef. Sushma was good at clearing (even to this day she's got a spotless kitchen), Hema at laying the table. My sisters also had to make Mum and Dad's bed in the morning. I was the cleaner of the bathrooms, then later the food serving girl.

Rajesh did nothing. Of course. Even back then I felt the injustice of that. Why were we girls slaving and he got to do precisely zero? Once we had prepared the meal, we all sat at the table together and Mum would always come to the table last or eat last – the food would always be cold by then. She always took the worst food, **'That roti, the one that got burnt, I'll eat it.'** And I'd think, Mum, don't eat the burnt roti. Why are you eating the old rice? But that was what was expected of her, and it had been instilled in her to care about herself and her needs last.

On Sundays, we would often go on some kind of adventure in the car. Dad loved a beauty spot, and we'd crisscross the country, taking the scenic routes to historic buildings and nature reserves. I still have little tableaux in my mind of Dad at Chatsworth House, sitting on a deckchair, taking in the view, regaling us with his knowledge of the 'magic violin door' that we'd just seen: a trompe l'oeil painting that certainly looked three-dimensional, with a violin that appeared to hang from a real metal peg. After Dad had explained it was an illusion, he managed to fall through his deckchair. All of us fell about in fits of giggles. Mum and me snorting with laughter and our customary unstoppable silent shaking.

Planning for one of these trips was like an army manoeuvre. Dad standing at the front door shouting instructions, flamboyantly dressed, no matter how inappropriate for being out in the countryside. His handkerchief matched his shirt, sticking out of his 'safari suit' pocket. He'd make sure everything fitted into the dark blue metallic Wolseley car.

I would describe him as precious because he never wanted to be late. If we were travelling by plane or train, if he could he would have made us camp the night before at the station for an early start. The same with any car journey: before the trip there were high levels of anxiety about whether we had enough time. Everybody would run around non-stop, getting things together for the long journey. Dad would shout orders and supervise the loading of the boot and roof rack. His booming voice became increasingly agitated: 'Hem, Sush, Shob, every one *chalo*, hurry up we are going to be late...'

Mum would be making sure everyone had gone to the bathroom and would complain that with all this running around the house we sounded like a herd of elephants. If a door slammed or if anything was knocked over, she would shout, **'What's dropped?'** What stays in my head is that no matter how many toilets we had in the house, we all wanted to use just the one. The blue bathroom – named because of the blue tiles and blue bathroom suite. I managed to dodge Dad on the landing and go to the downstairs cloakroom toilet. As ever, everyone ended up banging on the door for their coats.

Mum shouting, **'Shobi Shobi, *beti*, you are always the last, what are you doing in there? Have you shut the bathroom window? I don't know, you're always sitting on the toilet. Do you live there? Ha? Do you live there?'**

Mum would become more insistent. **'Get your brother's coat, he's outside already, he'll catch cold.'**

Every trip meant one of Mum's picnics. She would make up a large flask of curry – either potato or peas, definitely vegetarian for Mrs Health and Safety, so even if it was 'just' warm it wouldn't upset your tummy – and we'd soak it up with cold fried puris, rotis or double roti, depending on what we'd got left over. Everyone was somewhat nervous of carrying Mum's big red flask because it had glass inside – it had **'What did you do Shobna?'** written all over it. We were all sad when it finally broke as it could hold six portions of the mixed vegetable sabji in it – I can't remember if it was actually me, but I'm sure I got the blame for it.

The car journeys themselves were always epic, like the chariot race in *Ben-Hur* except without the other chariots. We always had to 'get there' with Dad in command of the steering wheel, Mum next to him with the Ordnance Survey map. We all piled in the back, me directly behind Dad, one bum cheek on the seat, the rest of me in the seat well. Raj in the middle and Sushma and Hema fighting over the passenger-side window seat. I knew it was best to be directly behind Dad because if I pissed him off I was always liable for a quick swipe, even if he was driving, and this way he couldn't reach me.

Hema would begin singing, which meant everyone had to join in. I was shy and I invariably didn't. Mum would often say I was 'painfully' shy and I can recall her telling my siblings to be quiet, **'Shobi's singing.'**

(When Mum asked once, **'Have you got everything you need in your little handbag?'** I responded, 'Where's me antiperspirant?' She found my Lancashire accent really amusing.)

My dad often wanted us to sing ABBA songs. He'd say, 'Sing "Chiquitita"'. It was one of his favourites. Hema would start the song, two octaves too high. Sushma would groan, 'That's too high, Hem!' and exclaim about how was she meant to join in or sing the harmony comfortably. Raj, loving the fun, would join in too, until the whole car was rocking out till we reached our destination.

Our family home's name of Geetanjali, which was displayed on a beautiful, handwritten-style sign outside, meant 'house of song', as my mother and father loved music. Dad believed this was something we could bring to our new home and it was one of the few parts of our cultural heritage we were totally encouraged to dip our toes into. He was the founder of the local Asian Arts Association, and with the Overseas Doctors Association he organized many cultural events. Singers, musicians and dancers gave classical concerts and they all stayed at our house. Our 'new extension', which had a large living room, would be in full swing with the sound of *ghazals*. Hema would sit cross-legged playing the Indian harmonium, morning to night, singing with Dad and you could catch Mum secretly humming along and dancing at the kitchen sink next door.

I started 'Indian dancing' at the age of seven. In contrast to my provocative behaviour at home, I was painfully shy outside it, and both my parents were keen for me to find 'my thing'. When I found it in the arts, I think they were so encouraging because it brought something out of me. Dancing was what really built my confidence and Dad arranged for a teacher of Sri Lankan heritage to conduct dance classes in his surgery when it was shut at the weekend. I really took to it then. When a bunch of other girls wanted to get involved too, we hired out the church hall and we learnt a variety of folk dances from across India, alongside Bharata Natyam, South Indian classical dance. Soon we started to perform what we had learnt. That's probably the first time Mum started to collect my little clippings – we did these events for our extended family and the local community as it grew.

Aside from dancing, my other way to be close to Mum was to go to the theatre with her. She loved it all – thrillers, farce, pantomimes, am-dram, any kind of English theatre. From the moment I could sit in a seat, I'd go with her and be her little girl, watching whatever it was she'd booked – and I absolutely loved it too. I would lose myself in the theatre and the stories and, just like Mum, I loved it all. Mum was so happy for me to be involved in the arts, so I took the extra drama classes in school and I was in all the plays, on the stage and backstage. Yes, I did adore it, but I wanted to please her more than anything. We were also all singers in the choir – we were basically the Indian von Trapp family. I have always carried around a half-remembered grain of a memory that once I was told that Gulati means somersault, and I like to think that in the past we were performers, a little like circus travellers, because every single one of us Gulatis had an urge to perform.

As well as school and chamber choirs, doing all the choral works, all the big school productions, Hema and Sushma were also in a pop band, which gave us bragging rights to being the trendiest Indian family in Oldham. The band was called The Golden Eagles and they did Bollywood, Beatles and Abba covers. There were three Gujarati boys from Ashton-under-Lyne on drums, guitar and electronic keyboard. They wore light brown safari suits and motorcycle-cop-style sunglasses, and Hema and Sushma were the lead singers. Mum made all their clothes – she either bought and adapted them or stitched them from scratch. She was always very methodical and loved sewing, so it was a creative outlet that suited her.

When my parents first arrived in Oldham there were just a few overseas doctors. But more people arrived, with new waves of immigration from Kenya and Uganda, as well as Pakistan and Bangladesh. For the northern towns it was a slow trickle, but gradually the community grew, so there were audiences for the band and for the dancing, and people started to make more connections with each other across the 'South Asian' communities. Different languages, religions, class and culture came together, bonded by a homogenous nostalgia for 'back home' and coupled with people's desire to reinterpret that into something that would reflect their present and future lives in the UK.

As my mother grew older and gained the confidence of a mother of four who had built a life on the other side of the world from her family, she gradually gained more independence. After many failed attempts, she passed her driving test, which gave her a new freedom (and my dad an excuse to buy another car). She also started secretly (not that Dad would have ever stopped her) to educate herself. Over time, the meekness she'd been raised with began to fade. As a young woman she had been a mix: a total force of nature and intimidating, but also submissive and docile as she tried to live up to what was expected of her as a wife. But she became many different women as she started to understand herself and the world around her more. She became an avid reader of the papers and listener of the *Today* programme. Her old Bush radio came to every new home and I remember her watching the news and drama on television constantly. She always tried to soak up more and more knowledge about the world.

Both my parents were politically engaged but they voted for different parties. Dad was a socialist to his core – he worked solidly and solely for the NHS, because he believed in it. That's one of the reasons he chose the UK, because he believed in health care for all. My mum, on the other hand, was at one time a mini Margaret Thatcher, mostly because she wanted to support a female politician. In India there was Indira Gandhi, in Pakistan there was Benazir Bhutto, and Mum, awakening as a feminist, felt it was the time for women to lead the world. She was proud of them and felt it her duty to support them.

I think Mum thought of herself as a bit of an Iron Lady: insular, strong, formidable. She'd always been quick-witted, perhaps to cover up the gaps in her knowledge. Now that she'd started fill those gaps, her inner compass was shifting and with it the balance at home.

This led to a lot of debates in the house. When my sisters were old enough to vote, out the front of our house there were three different boards: 'Vote Conservative!' 'Vote Labour!' and 'Vote Liberal!' Blue, red and yellow. Luckily Mum's time as a Tory supporter didn't last too long, once she realized Thatcher's real political agenda.

My mum believed deeply in sincerity, it was one of the guiding values of her life. She had a very solid morality and her ideas of what was right were unshakeable. With my mother's growing sense of self and formation of her own beliefs and moral judgements came a lot of fights. The arguments were about people Dad had brought into their lives that Mum felt were false and disingenuous, or sometimes the arguments centred on his partying or playing golf. My dad lived fast, my mum lived slow. After one argument about my father drinking and smoking, the accusations still hanging above both their heads, my mother took out all his cigars and smoked every single one of them in front of him, then poured herself a lager and added a Rose's lime cordial top.

Despite the rows, my father was very open to her opinions, always encouraging her to follow her ideas and allowing her to develop them, which was fairly unusual for a North Indian husband. She could push things further because the boundaries were designed not to be too tight. As with their love, their lives could stretch out unconditionally to fit each other within them.

CHAPTER TWO

What is wrong with you?

Growing up, *I* was a problem.

By night, my parents deconstructed their day with one another. Their bedroom was next to mine, with thin walls dividing us, so I would listen to their interchanging whispers. I was often the subject of their pillow talks via a high drama monologue from my mum:

'She just doesn't know when to stop.'

'What have I done to deserve this?'

'She is killing me!' (The sound of a muffled thud of her hand hitting her chest.)

'What will I do?'

'Day in day out...Hai!'

'Who will ever want her?'

'If she doesn't eat, she will die...if she dies, I will die, Hai

Ram Hai Ram...'

Then a curt response from Dad: 'Well, she's YOUR daughter... turn the light off, darling.' The sound of the pull of the light cord above their bed.

'She must be suffering from "third child syndrome"', my dad's tired voice offered, minutes later.

Tucked up in my bed, listening to my parents' conversation, I was totally convinced that whatever I was 'suffering from' appeared to be terminal.

Mornings in our household were always chaos – children and parents running up and down the same stairs, near collisions on the landing between the two different sets of steps. Plenty of shouting, thudding about and in-fighting. Mum would be forcing the last spoon of milk-laden cereal into my reluctant 13-year-old mouth (no matter how old I was, if I didn't eat, I was fed), scraping the cereal bowl with vigour, another one of her monologues punctuated with the sound of the very large round spoon, banging the sides of the bowl for further emphasis:

'I don't know why you don't eat.' (Bang.)

'How old are you, ha?' (Bang.)

I would wait for the next clatter of the spoon or *ha*. (The ha was simply rhetorical.) Questioning my every move or motive for my behaviour. A bang of the spoon and then:

'Starving?... yes, you look like a famine victim, thi chacha laga. Daddy is already in the car, Sushma and Hema doing the beds...and you? You sit here like a camel.'

My cheeks, full of food.

My brother skipping out of the kitchen, after finishing his breakfast 'like a good boy'. I was convinced I could hear 'THE BOY' applause every time he moved.

I would pray that Mum would get distracted and not notice that I hadn't drunk my milk. After force-feeding me cereal till the bowl was spotless, she would take out her frustration by thoroughly rinsing all the utensils, bowls, plates, pots and pans till they were meticulously clean before they went into the dishwasher. That was part of her 'cleaning up' theory which has remained a complete enigma to me to this day.

I'd wait till Mum went into the front room to start the prep for my next problematic trait – my unruly hair – making sure the comb, hairbrush and regulation school uniform coloured bobbles were at the ready. In the kitchen, I would quickly spit out my food and then clean the sink to hide any evidence.

In the living room I'd stand mutely in front of her, trying hard to make no sound at all as Mum plaited my hair. Mum had to rush, and she hated being rushed, but Dad would never tolerate being late for work and he took us to school in the mornings. If I ever complained as she combed through the knots, grumbling about 'this bird's nest' at the back of my head, she would threaten me with a short back and sides.

Once my hair was completed, her face would look softer. She'd turn up the radio for 'Thought for the Day', scheduled just before the 8am news, and I would grab my packed lunch and hotfoot it out of the house. I was always the last into the car, as the radio bips sounded and the headlines were read. Then Mum's face would poke out of the front doorway just as I was about to slam the car door shut, making sure she had the last word:

'**Shobi, Shobi I know that you haven't had your milk! What? Is that what you're doing? Teaching your grandmother to suck eggs, ha? Two cups of Ovaltine, when you get home after school...thi chacha laga hurry up, challo challo.**'

My heart would sink, as I knew when I got home after school

my original cup of Ovaltine would still be waiting for me, the skin of the milk congealed on the top, alongside another hot cup. Nothing could ever or would ever be wasted. Milk was 'good for me' and I needed feeding up.

I didn't get my period until I was about 14 and up until that point I hadn't developed a woman's body at all. There was another girl at swimming club called Samantha and Mum always said to me, **'Why don't you look like that? Samantha has a perfect neat figure, she looks like a woman, you look like a boy.'** How the bloody hell would I know? Did she not know how frustrated I was by my lack of female development?

One day, I found blood in my pants. As the third daughter you'd think I would have been prepared, but nothing had ever been mentioned. I ran to my mum to tell her what had happened and she replied, cool as you like, **'Yes darling, that's your womb breaking down.'** Then not a single other word was said. I can recall thinking, My what? My womb? Where is that?

We weren't allowed tampons. In fact, I didn't use a tampon until I went to university (the freedom!). All I knew was that Mum had a box of Kotex pads in the bathroom cupboard, and if you bled you used one and then packed the box away. You put the pad in the bin after use, wrapped in old newspaper, and made sure no one saw anything, not a trace of it. I had no idea when Mum had a period or was going through the menopause. I never once spoke to my sisters about it either. It wasn't a women's shared secret, it was your own secret shame to keep to yourself and clear up, as if it had never happened. Nothing like that was ever spoken about. (At least sanitary towels were better than what I would later use in India. When I was 16 living with my naniji, she made me pack down old cotton rags and wash and dry them in the back yard every day of my period.)

On top of no tampons, Mum banned us from removing any hair. Pubic hair, leg hair, underarm hair, eyebrows, moustaches, all of it. She said it would just grow back thicker so we shouldn't do it. I'm sure she was right, but I was a little furball. So I gave up swimming because I couldn't remove my leg hair or my underarm hair, which had grown even if my boobs and hips hadn't. I looked like a pubescent boy, unlike Samantha. I also have a massive birthmark on my right hip which I used to try and cover by putting my hand over it – but there's only so much a hand can cover. As for make-up? We weren't allowed that either.

I can remember being in bed in my early teens, my hands placed at the top of my folded-down sheet, the tips of my fingers catching the top of the soft grey blanket. I was all tucked up in my single bunk bed, now slotted into two white chipboard slats; on one side was the MDF wardrobe, on the other the dressing table and mirror. The wallpaper, patterned with a picture of a girl and boy holding hands and grinning, was peeling slightly, and a round brass frame displayed a small Polynesian girl with a multicoloured garland of flowers around her neck. She was a neat-featured, pretty girl, and had the biggest black eyes in the whole world. How I wished that she was my own reflection. Mum stood in the doorway of my room. Her beautiful figure silhouetted by the night lamp in the corridor. Her voice soft and authoritative, **'Shobna, where are your hands?'**

I wiggled my fingers defiantly to show her exactly where they were. Mum went downstairs and I counted her every step until I knew she was in the TV room. Then quick as a flash I turned on my side and put my hands between my thighs, just above my knees.

I had no idea why she was asking. In hindsight, she must have been checking to see if I was masturbating – it was the furthest thing from my mind.

As a child, before we had a shower installed, bathing always involved mixing hot water into buckets with cold water, and sitting in an empty, cold bath. It was always straight in and straight out of these bucket baths, being wrapped quickly in a towel, then dressing in radiator-warmed clothes, no hanging about whilst you were naked or even in covered in your towel – that would never be tolerated. *Sharam*, the concept of shame, had been integral to our lives. We had all been brought up to be ashamed of our very bodies. A peek of skin would prompt a song from Mum about the shame of nudity: **'Shame, shame, poppy shame, all the monkeys know your name.'**

On one family holiday in Sweden, in the changing rooms after swimming, Mum was horrified at the Swedes' attitude surrounding nudity. She would marvel at the women, and say, **'They're putting on their lipstick before they're putting on their clothes?'** Modesty was key for the girls in the house and we had to make sure that we respected our differences from the men of the house and kept separate. My friends at school told stories of family holidays where brothers and sisters all together would bathe with no shame. I remember being totally gobsmacked. In our household being naked in front of anybody else was wrong, and we were all incredibly self-conscious and embarrassed by our bodies.

Where had this been instilled into my parents? Was it a lasting legacy of the Victorians in India? We never asked any questions though, we just followed the rules. This has led to me feeling, throughout my adult life, very shy about being nude. Indeed, years later, my mother accidentally ran into me as I came out of her en-suite shower, naked. Looking me up and down, she gestured towards the meeting of my thighs and said, with a questioning hand, **'What is that? Fashion?'**

It probably comes as no surprise that in the Gulati household there was absolutely no conversation around sex. As far as I knew, my life's plan was as follows: I would meet a suitable boy and I would be married off to him. Sex would then 'occur'. I would have loved to know more about sex. More than just the diagrams in biology class. I'm from that first generation of sex education, where we had extremely graphic sex-ed books, but no one came away from the late 1970s sex-ed much the wiser. I didn't understand how babies were made, despite the pictures in those books and our embarrassed chatter in the girls' cloakroom at school.

Back then, studying was my life, because if I didn't study, I was useless. I wanted to just fit in and please everyone. But at a certain point, that was going to change.

My father's educational motto was 'you have to be *so much* better than everybody else, because when an examiner sees your name, they will know you aren't white'. Underlying this was the assumption that the examiner would mark us harder as we weren't one of them. We were to give them no excuses to penalize us for being 'foreigners'. He knew this only too well, as his desire to become a consultant had been thwarted by institutionalized racism. He had a family to support and our school fees to pay and the fight had proved harder than the reward. He had weighed up the consequences of his ambition and decided to ultimately leave his dream behind, becoming a GP instead, but he always made sure that we knew to do our best and he hoped we would beat the system.

My school was the local grammar – The Hulme Grammar School for Girls – and both my sisters had gone there before me. Hema was very popular and responsible and was voted deputy head girl. Sushma was also well-known in the school, she was in the pop band and everything. She had also developed the most amazing hourglass figure. She, too, became deputy head girl. Then there was me.

I was a very boyish, goth/emo girl (I loved wearing black and listening to very moody music) who sat in her bedroom all the time and was painfully shy outside of the family's four walls. I had a special group of friends – we were all outsiders and very awkward. But I still maintained that ability to be everything to everyone, and sometimes even the more popular girls would allow me into their group. Still, I was surprised that I, too, became deputy head girl – in hindsight I suspect the school didn't want to break our family tradition.

My school was attached to the boys' grammar. There was a glass door that divided the two, and aside from glimpses through the gaps in the curtain that covered it, for most of my teenage years I lived in a gender apartheid. I had a succession of mad crushes on both girls and boys. My first male crush was for one of the teachers at the boys' school and then I had another one on a teacher's son. I never did anything about any of it, I just swooned from afar. Or scrawled their names on my rough copy book with a series of love hearts and kisses, alongside an array of pop stars and Manchester United footballers cut out and pasted onto the front and back covers.

Although I was allowed to speak to boys (as I was the third daughter, lots of the battles surrounding accessibility to boys had already been hard-won by my sisters), I was completely sheltered from what a relationship could actually involve. It wasn't so much that I was *prevented* from, say, having sex, it was more that I was totally unaware of what it was. All I knew was that you could be disowned by your parents if you 'went too far with a boy' but beyond that lay a great expanse of unknown that I had no interest in trespassing into.

But I did want to fall in love. Love was something I could understand as it was a quotidian aspiration of my peers and my sisters and, after all, my mum and dad were the most loving couple. They were our role models. Aged 18, I met a boy at a conference organized by the Overseas Doctors' Association in Middleton and I instantly fell in love. He was from Romford in Essex, and after that first meeting we struck up a pen-pal relationship. We wrote letters and letters and letters and letters and letters. It's no wonder my schoolwork suffered, as I devoted hours to writing reams to him:

> I made the sun shine though it wasn't, by thinking about you. Even though you're not physically near, you are there helping me all the way. I love you and I'm sorry about the burst of emotion on t'phone on Thurs. Though it certainly helped, I feel great now and ready to work as hard as I can coz I want everything to work out hunky-dory for us. You deserve it to work out and I'm gonna make it work out wiv you so we're gonna do it together. I want to hug you right now and tell you just how much I need you. Yes, I've jumped in with both my feet as it were. I love you so much that my insides want to burst. You're no heartache you're my happiness, my inspiration.

(That's only page 2 of 10!)

They were full of teenage angst, escapist thoughts and wants, and discussions around our shielded culture. What is startling is that I was a legal adult, but I was still so naive. The theme that remains constant throughout these epistles was whether we would ever be alone together. Could we go to go to the cinema together? Could we go for food together? Could it just be him and me?

Then there was a boy at school I used to hang out with sometimes, and a third boy that I'd met at a family party who used to take me to galleries. My father would laugh about it. He'd say, 'You've got one on the phone, one is writing letters and one is on the drive ringing the doorbell. What to do, *ay*?' He felt I spent too much time and energy on the phone 'talking to boys', telling me that I needed to prioritize my education and grades. Also, making 'long distance' calls in the day and not after 6pm, for hours on end, was costing him a small fortune.

It's true that I always had more than one boyfriend on the go, as I was never going to be exclusive with a boy who didn't want to commit to being in a proper girlfriend/boyfriend relationship with me, like the ones I'd seen in my sister's *Jackie* magazines. I wasn't having any full-on sexual dalliances, so that wasn't the issue. I just liked the different company and exploring this new world of boys. This attitude was perhaps surprising as I'm an Indian girl and, in their stereotype, I'm supposed to be trapped by my cultural patriarchy. But this development distanced me from my dad. As new male figures began to march into my mind, my focus on my father and obtaining his praise drifted off. Men weren't just fathers, they were also people my own age and my attention was all theirs.

It's surprising that boys were at all interested in me as I'd also gone from being a cutesy kid to looking extremely awkward. My mum would tell me that Indian girls' noses had to grow to reach the sun in this country because the weather was so terrible – and she made no bones about how big mine was becoming. Cruelly, Mum's nose was a very delicate princess shape which made me more aware of the size of my own. I was also skinny, without any semblance of a woman's figure at all. Looking back at me from the mirror was hair, limbs, no bum, with a big nose and joined-up eyebrows. My sisters called me 'Man-chester' as I had 'two fried eggs for breasts'.

As a family we were supposed to be presentable and neat, and nothing I could do would make me either. I was all at odds with my growing body. My father was also a very flashy man who wanted us all to be glitzy and glamorous, so whenever we went anywhere he would tell me to wear heels and get out of my black oversized second-hand goth attire. But true to my nickname of Little Miss Controversy, I would rebel and be called out as *zidi* (stubborn). Still, though, being brainy was ultimately more important than being attractive, so despite my 'limp' hair, sometimes I got away with it.

The things I loved at school were all focused on stories. I was so good at making them up. As a very young child, my make-believe tales had included living in India in a hut with snakes, and telling my open-mouthed friends at school the fantastical tale of how Dad had bored a hole in my mum's head with a bradawl and filled it with coloured powder to indicate 'she's my woman', when I'd got bored of explaining for the thousandth time why she wore a bindi. I'd also told stories of how my parents were so strict about our studying that I was tied to a chair by the table to make me concentrate. It's a wonder social services didn't turn up!

But nothing hooked me as much as dancing. I certainly never felt freer, even within the rigid, classical structure of Indian dance. I had continued to go to see all the Asian Arts Association programmes with Mum, and when I was about ten, I watched Chitra Visweswaran dance who crystallized everything for me. She was so gymnastic and vigorous, expressing the more masculine *tandav* style, then at another point she was softer, moving in a curve pattern dance, storytelling through gesture and facial expressions in a *lasya*, more female style of dance. She inhabited these movements and characters with such clarity. The fact that one body, this one particular woman's body, was capable of such strength and grace gave me a desperate urge to learn this new way of being and moving.

Immediately after I finished my O levels, I'd flown to Delhi to study dance at my naniji's house. I was lucky enough to have a teacher who taught me the Bharata Natyam in a very strict way and to a very high standard. In my mind, that was it – I was never going back to school. It wasn't a hobby any more to bring me out of my shell; it was my reason to be.

In fact, during that time I spent in India, my naniji had made 'introductions' for me. I remember one called Bunkim Bunkim – so good they named him twice! She'd said, 'Shobna, *beti*, put a nice shalwar kameez on,' and I said, 'Naniji, what am I going to do when I'm married and I go and make him a cup of tea in the morning? Do I shout Bunkim Bunkim...Bunkim, breakfast is ready...?'

Nani laughed so hard she spat out a little round potato she had been eating. When he later came round to the house for high tea you could see she was shaking trying not to laugh as I dutifully offered him a china cup of freshly brewed tea on a matching saucer and a hot samosa. Afterwards she enquired whether I liked him. I said, 'Well, he had nice feet.' To which she added, 'Well, that's something, better than nothing, *hai na*?'

Then she introduced me to a young man who worked for Cadbury's India. I called him Willy Wanker, because his family had decided I was too 'western' and therefore I was 'fast'. What an unfair judgement and how far from my reality. You see, it was in India and not in the 'fast west', I had my first real initiation into the world of men and women. I was 16 going on 17 when a boy first took his penis out in front of me. We had gone to the cinema that summer of all my suitable boy introductions, and he got it out in the middle of the movie and asked me to touch it. I thought, What?! Why would I want to do that?

'Please put it back where it came from,' I said politely. I had never seen one in real life and I was totally grossed out by him.

But then all my dreams of India ended suddenly. In the middle of a class, I was being reprimanded by my *guruji* (teacher) – he had told me to make my 'y'elbows less curved and more straightaaaaa', but not that straight as I was quite tall and limby, it was my body shape that was his frustration – when my father phoned to tell me I'd got all nine of my O levels, but 'only' got five As, and I had to come back to do my A levels.

I threw a big tantrum about it and tried to put my foot down, but he sent my uncle over from Mumbai to convince me that I had no choice. I remember my uncle telling me that I'd end up prostituting myself on some Bollywood casting couch if I didn't go home. They were very traditional and I had little power to assert myself. I was, of course, in their eyes, simply a girl. So I put my dancing career on hold, despite how accomplished I had become, and stepped back into the restricted contours of education.

My grades and performance in school were enough for me to be invited for an interview at Cambridge for Robinson College and Mum drove me down. The only thing I can really remember about the trip was us polishing off a full English breakfast at our lovely B&B, then wrapping up the extras in tissues and stowing them in her bag for later – and indeed, on the way home, she offered me the saved food. Aside from the aptitude test and interview at Cambridge, I also interviewed at SOAS (the School of Oriental and African Studies), because I really wanted to study Hindi and Sanskrit (which would conveniently sit alongside any extra curricular Indian classical dance study) and both universities offered me conditional places with grades that were well within my reach.

When the phone rang in the early hours of 11 January 1985, I woke up to its ring reverberating off the walls. Whenever we got a call in the early hours, we always knew it meant something had happened in India, and that it would be something terrible.

My father was visiting India, so it was my mother who answered the phone. It's her voice that I remember most clearly, saying, '**Sacmuc? Sacmuc? Sacmuc?**' Really? Really? Really?

I knew something unbelievable must have happened when I heard sobs replace her words, and my stomach dropped.

Mum called Hema, who came running from her bedroom on the far side of the house. I could hear them both crying.

She had been told that her husband had died in his sleep. In the same bed in India I had slept in a year or so before.

For such a momentous juncture, my recollections of that time are shattered into fragments, slivers of memories which I've never been able to reassemble into anything that could form a whole memory again. As though it couldn't hold on to the sheer weight of what was happening and the change that had suddenly ripped through our lives.

Dad had been staying at my naniji's in New Delhi, organizing things for my sister Hema's *rishta* (marriage proposal), as she was to have an arranged marriage later that year. He had been sorting her trousseau, saris and jewellery that could only be bought in India. Mum had stayed home with Raja and me, because we were both in school.

The day Dad had left our house to fly to India, we'd had another argument over my phone use and the boy in Romford. Dad had met him by this point, because he was starting to seem like a more serious prospect, and all the family thought that he was going to become a firm fixture in my life. But Dad thought my boyfriend was the reason I wasn't revising and he was really very angry with me.

All I could think about is how pleased I was that they were all going to the airport to see Dad off, as it would mean I would have the house all to myself so I could call my boyfriend back in peace. My mum had come into my room with her look – the look that said, you are going to do exactly what I tell you to – and she said that Dad was at the door and she wanted me to go and say goodbye and make up. Begrudgingly I did.

I don't know how it would have been if I hadn't said goodbye. I gave him another hug, then went to walk back in when I heard him shout out: 'Hem, Sush, Sho. Hem, Sush, Sho.' This time I went back to the door for a hug and to promise I'd revise and that I'd get to Cambridge. Then he left and I never saw him again.

Dad was such a pillar of society, so very popular and comprehensively loved all across the local community – he'd broken through social and cultural divides, as well as colour prejudice. Everybody suddenly descended on our doorstep and wanted to get involved. The house was full of people, every uncle and aunty in disbelief at this news. Because he died abroad, Oldham Parish Church opened its doors so that everyone in the local community could pay their respects. Still today people remind me that I'm 'Dr Gulati's daughter'.

My dad was only 49. My mother and father and all of us had celebrated their silver wedding anniversary the previous November – a glittering occasion in a local council hall, entertainment by all the Gulati von Trapp. We all sang, I gave a classical dance performance and my brother played tabla. Mum and Dad discoed into the night surrounded by three hundred or so of their friends. Mum wearing a super-glamorous midnight blue sari with a white and gold embroidered border and Dad in a light blue suit. Forever dancing in shades of blue with one another against the backdrop of a twinkling starry sky stage curtain.

Back at the house, Mum was there physically, but emotionally it was like she had dissolved into the crowd – it felt like I couldn't reach her. Then doctors came in with all these tranquillizers. We were all hysterical.

They gave me pills too.

In among this mist, Mum, Hema and Raja left to go India.

I stayed behind as I had my A level mocks. Sushma had important exams at dental school too. The decision was taken that I should be kept in a controlled environment, and I went to live with family friends in Rochdale. I couldn't tell you how long I was there for, but I had no contact at all with Mum or my siblings while they were away. Nothing. I was suddenly alone without my family for support.

I later found out that Dad had had an open funeral pyre and that my 14-year-old brother had to deal with the last rites. He found it a culture shock: funeral pyres on the Ganges were what we watched on television documentaries. The Hindu ritual of my dad's death in Benares (now Varanasi) was far removed from our experience of the sanitized and clinical western culture of cremation.

At some point they flew back and I went home. The house felt completely different. Everything was so quiet, so sedate, so solemn. Dad had been a ball of full-on energy and everything spinning around him had been high drama; he had lit the rooms from within. His name, Kulbhushan, means 'the centre of the family' and our centre had been hollowed out.

It was a feeling of loss beyond losing my father, a loss of what had been, now irrevocably gone from us all. Our flamboyant, dynamic household; my parents entwined at parties, always so close to each other; friends coming in and out of the door; 'Hem, Sush, Sho, Hem, Sush, Sho' booming up and down the stairs.

Life had been a constant *clink clink* celebration, with my sisters singing in the background, me dancing, applause following my brother everywhere he went for growing into the handsome and clever young man my family had so longed for. Then it collapsed in one night. All of it over. The grief inside our house so desperate and intense that I could feel its pressure pushing on my chest, everything so tight, ready to burst and fill this dark expanse we were left with.

My mum still kept up her Monday fast for a long time after Dad's death. As part of Punjabi tradition during the festival of Karva Chauth, she would drive around, dressed up in full 'out out' sari, bedecked, bejewelled and 'bindied' (after Dad's death she stopped wearing a bindi), searching the cloudy skies for the concealed moon. I'd be in the car with her with a *katori* (small bowl) of water, a lit candle and a sieve (although today, I'm still trying to decipher the significance of the sieve). These were all tools for her to perform the ritual of breaking her fast when we finally spotted the auspicious moon. Once my dad died, her dress for this and every other occasion became more subdued, but she kept up this observance and devotion, even though it hadn't prevented Dad from dying before his time. She would ask, **'What have I done to deserve this?'** to which I wish I had answered, 'You didn't do anything wrong. You always did your absolute best.'

I can only describe life at this stage as watching the colour seep from the walls. As though we had all been living in Technicolour and suddenly it faded and bleached out to monochrome. A reversed *Wizard of Oz*. Our mother's vibrant-coloured clothes disappeared as Hindu widows are expected to shun bright shades. In the strictest communities they are supposed to wear white until they die, existing in a permanent state of mourning. I always think of how much my mum loved her bindis. She'd had all these little boxes and I can remember rifling through them, stacked like the spices in picture books of faraway souks in fairy tales, these pigmented powders in incandescent purples, reds, magentas and oranges. Using her tiny, very ornate, metal moulds, she'd made big or small rounds and stick them on with Nivea cream. You'd spot tiny flecks of rainbow-shaded dust on her nose. Like her scent (her favourite was Estée Lauder's Youth Dew) and her immaculate hair, it was something inimitably her. That little ritual was a daily joy to her, but after my father died it was not permitted.

Mum was only 45 when Dad died and was a fine-looking woman, and none of us wanted her to be shrouded in white. I think of myself at her age – I was in the prime of my womanhood and I can't imagine what it would have been like to have to adopt these restrictive modes of dressing. The deep colours from her wardrobe disappeared, much like how her character withdrew, suddenly only to be found in the shadows. She had been muted.

CHAPTER THREE

Do you think I don't know my daughter?

In among this shrouded period of my life, my exams took place. They didn't go as planned and I didn't achieve the results I needed for Cambridge. They were enough for me to still attend SOAS, but at that point I felt emotionally bereft. So much of my education had been focused on my father, measured by him and committed to please him, and now he was gone. I didn't want to be hundreds of miles away from family, from Mum, so I applied to Manchester University through clearing, as did my boyfriend from Romford, and we both got our places.

We would live in student accommodation. This would give us freedom from our family homes, and the chance to be a proper couple, which would hopefully lead to us getting married. Mum told me that the day I left to go off to university with my boyfriend, I smiled for the first time since Dad died – my face was filled with the brightness a fresh start promised. Like the ancient Greek phoenix, I was ready to rise from the ashes of our burnt-down world. There was hope and it was beginning to steal its way back into my person.

Things had changed for my family now my dad was gone. In the community, a husband provided all the women in his family protection, and within a few weeks of his death it became clear our buffer against the world had vanished. My boyfriend's mother came to visit us that summer before we went to university and expressed her disapproval of the match. She brought a male family friend with her – as her husband was working abroad, she needed a man to accompany her for validation – knowing full well my mum would be alone. She said that she'd read my letters and found them to be too sexual in content. The contents of these 'lewd' letters centred on my expressing that I wanted us to be together and, when that time came, how we would make it special; how other boys at school did not see me as a person but wanted just to 'go all the way'; how my ex-'friend' at school had been a bit too pushy and how I was ashamed of that. With strict eyes I could be seen as a little forward, but it was hardly offensive. I hadn't *done* anything shameful.

His mum intimated that I was some northern hussy trying to trap her son with pregnancy. But the underlying truth is that the conversation wouldn't have happened if Dad had still been there; as a widowed family, we were now vulnerable and exposed. Similarly, Hema didn't marry her fiancé. After my dad's passing, her soon-to-be in-laws suddenly demanded that Mum pay to redecorate their kitchen as part of Hema's dowry. It had also transpired that this not-such-a-gentleman already had an English girlfriend on the go and didn't really want to get married at all. And so the future unions of my sister and me unravelled, just as our collective family unit had done when my father died (though for me, I did not know at that point that my relationship would eventually falter).

One of the difficulties was that our father had been very progressive, and he was a big advocate of assimilation as one of the first post-Empire children to properly settle in England. But as the North Indian Punjabi community in Britain grew over the years, it became more rigid and exacting with its rules on what was right and wrong. What was Indian tradition and what was not. What was allowed and what was not. It was as though each of these families had to hold on to their traditions with a vice-like grip for fear they might lose themselves and their cultural 'identity'.

India was moving on with the times, but the Punjabi community in Britain had brought the past with them and clung on to it. Dad's open-minded attitudes had shielded us and allowed us to grow, he'd been in a position to push back and we were enfranchised in the fullest sense of the word . In contrast, once he was gone, our mother was 'just' a woman. In some quarters of this culture, without a man you're seen as nothing, therefore there is a sense that you no longer deserve any of the respect afforded to others. And my newly widowed mum was now confronted with this patriarchal order in all its forms.

It was at this time that I left my mother and my family home. I left her grief and the grief that encircled the house and had crept into every corner of it. I left the pressure I had felt weighing down on me for all those months, which needed to be released. I went completely off the rails.

My studies were not the place to escape and I lost myself

to drugs and alcohol and let my sadness be eaten up by them instead. It was the late 1980s, the height of excess. I smoked a lot of cannabis, which is not so great when you have to learn and conjugate 201 Arabic verbs. And while I started university in a relationship, I didn't end it in one. My boyfriend, it transpired, was relentlessly jealous and our time together left a huge imprint on me that remains to this day. The reason why I have all my letters to him is because he gave them all back. The relationship was not a happy one, I felt like I was constantly walking on eggshells and, looking back, it was a truly heinous experience.

Whenever I came home from university to visit my mother, I noticed that little things were changing. Our housekeeper, who had helped organize everything around the house, had passed around the same time as Dad. Mum still cleaned everything to within an inch of its life, she was looking after my brother and she was still very house-proud, but piles of newspapers started to build up. Elsewhere in the house, empty boxes that had previously been hidden out of sight (Mum and Dad habitually collected empty appliance boxes ready to be filled with their new stuff, just in case they were ever going to return to India) had started to accumulate in the corners of now-unused rooms, alongside plastic bags full of waste paper. It was as though she wanted to keep everything as it was as a way of blanketing herself from loss.

She had begun to give Nazar, or the 'evil eye', particular importance in her life and consequently in our lives too. In my mum's view, if we looked good or did particularly well at school, we would surely be on our way to rack and ruin as Nazar would get us and something terrible would befall us. Nazar would also create a space for anyone with malignant designs or who held jealousy or envy, which ultimately was properly shit for any good luck or blessings. So if someone looked good, Mum would say, **'You look horrible'**, and if she looked good, which she invariably did, we'd tell her we'd never seen her so ugly. All was said with a wink of an eye, and this way Nazar would be defeated and nothing bad would happen.

I've often thought about Mum's attachment to Nazar, and her consequent fear of how her beautiful life could suddenly be taken away from her if she ever allowed herself too much celebration. Her ideal partnership with the man she loved? Her complete and beautiful family? Maybe it had all been too much good fortune and now Nazar had crept in after her husband's death and this was all retribution, some kind of terrible 'poetic justice'.

My relationship with Mum was still there, but we weren't part of each other's day to day. I had become withdrawn and detached. I didn't really like my new university life. And although I visited fairly often, as I was only in Manchester I never stayed over. We never strayed beyond superficial conversation and I wasn't honest at all about my cannabis use or alcohol or boys. I wasn't open about my emotions or my feelings to any degree.

As a young person coming from the household I came from, the freedoms at university had been a baptism of fire. It goes without saying that any relationships where sex might have been involved were complicated to discuss. If it happened, you just didn't talk about it. The story is: you get married and you are allowed to have sex. If you told the real story to your parents, you'd be disowned. I had seen that happen to some girls from our community peer group and to a dear family friend who 'came out'. These were close family friends whose parents had completely repudiated their children in the most harmful of ways. You learn to keep quiet.

I had two different boyfriends at university and I kept very quiet about anything that happened with either of them. The interesting thing is, I don't really remember ever having had sex during that time. I felt entirely removed from my body. The edges of everything still felt so blurred, as though I didn't exist as a whole person. I wasn't ready for relationships…I knew what the blueprint was, but I had never been schooled in how to approach it. My parents only knew what they had experienced with each other, but that didn't fit with my reality and I had no emotional tools to deal with these relationships.

The only time Mum ever tried to touch on these taboo topics was in her car, when I was held captive – but instead of lecturing me on sex before marriage (as she would never consider talking about this) she asked me if I was gay. **'There must be something wrong with you. Two failed relationships with nice Indian boys already, and not even out of university.'**

After my degree, I decided I was going to finally pursue dancing, and now no one was going to stop me. I'd done my A levels, got my degree. I'd done what had been expected of me. Now I could finally be a dancer. I auditioned at the Laban Centre in London, got in and, a few weeks later, moved into a flat with a female barrister in Forest Hill with just a suitcase and my first boyfriend's teddy bear.

Mum said she was excited for me, and I believed her. After all, it had been Mum who had invested in my dancing with the teachers, ferrying me about to classes in her car, sewing costumes, paying for lessons and organizing dance events for all those years. But we didn't tell anyone in the community exactly what I was doing down in London – as far as they knew I had gone to do an arts administration course because I didn't want them to give Mum any more abuse about her 'free' daughters. People would smile and shake our hands but talk behind our backs, that's the way the community is.

During the year's course at Laban, I encountered microaggressions and blatant racial prejudice for the first time in my adult life. Junior school had been a place where I was the only 'Paki', to be roughed up in a game of British Bulldog. Every time we played, I was invariably the last one at the end of the pitch and then, to get to the other side, had to run through at least fifty kids, each of whom would want to take me down by any means necessary. My explanations for my knocked-out baby teeth and bruises were designed to shield my parents – 'I'd been climbing a tree' or 'I tripped over'.

Later, at the posh prep school, there was talk of my full lips being 'wog' lips – at which I now laugh, as some women have ended up with terrible trout pouts from lip-plumping procedures in their quest for beauty. My lips, just like my Black sisters', were beautiful all along. But at the time I didn't feel that way and I picked at them so badly I made them bleed as I played their hatred over in my mind. I didn't want to be different, no child does. By senior school, I was experiencing a less actively aggressive, yet still deliberately exclusory, form of racism, as I wasn't invited to some parties and was excluded from popular groups and teams. My university years passed me by in a haze. If anything had happened I was too deeply buried in my grief to notice.

By the time I got to Laban, I'd been told I made everything look 'Indian', that I moved like an Indian. I was informed that my dance background wasn't really technically classical, like ballet, it was 'folk'. I was viewed as an anthropological study and so was my art form. I felt like an exhibit in a theatrical zoo. An 'uncivilized', 'non-classical' 'storyteller'. Something to be looked down upon and not celebrated as high art. That's all any form of non-western dance could be in their eyes. Teachers told me that my alignment was problematic. I had become quite heavy-breasted and my posture suffered. My eating deteriorated. I was once told by a fellow student that I 'smelled of curry all the time'.

Then the dancer and choreographer Shobana Jeyasingh came to Laban to teach an Indian dance module and finally there was something that I got. And I was really good at it. One of my first jobs was to join her company, and I soon also started to work at the London Contemporary Dance Theatre at The Place (the renowned Bloomsbury-based dance space) and had the opportunity to learn about contemporary and 'new' dance at its crucible. I got deeply into the scene and began running workshops and teaching as well as dancing in theatre productions and in events. I had started to make a living in the arts.

One event was seminal – the French bicentenary celebrations in 1989 choreographed by Jean-Paul Goude (who, incidentally, was married to Grace Jones, my idol). The 'Défilé' processed down the Champs-Élysées in Paris and his vision was to include all the countries that had contributed to the creation of France, celebrating them in a worldwide festival of dance and culture. For Britain he wanted a host of Classical Indian dancers and a troupe of contemporary dancers. As a metaphor for Empire and India's place as the 'Jewel in the Crown', the white men of the contemporary dance group were dressed in military uniform and each held an umbrella over an Indian dancer, protecting us from the 'rain' created by the Kent Fire Brigade, who sprayed water on us as we danced our way down the Champs-Élysées. Jean-Paul added that the hosepipe water spray was apt because, 'it always rains in England'. After meeting me, he sent me off to the provincial towns to find '20 Shobnas' for the project, which I duly did. I organized auditions across Britain and found 20 young women of the 'like'.

That whole experience in France blew my mind, working away

for the first time and among all these people. It was really also
my first time recognizing my own sexuality in terms of choices.
Suddenly, I was open enough to consider a relationship with a
man or a woman, it didn't make a difference. It was the first time
I'd really seen people from all walks of life and backgrounds,
up close and personal. I was within a company of dancers and
performers who all seemed so confident in their bohemian and
liberated lifestyles. Yes, this liberation had been there at dance
school and at university, but I'd never been a part of it because I'd
been made to feel like an outsider. But in Paris, the gay and lesbian
scene hit me with a palpable force. It was the freedom of it all:
multi-partnered, bisexual people were experimenting with gender
and were entirely free to choose how they lived their lives. I was
intoxicated by this. And everything seemed to *finally* make sense.
It felt like I learnt everything I possibly could about life, choices,
gender and sexuality in that moment, but of course these kinds
of experiences were taking me further and further away from
the young woman my parents and the wider family had hoped
I would be. Although my mother had accepted that I'd gone on
another journey, she didn't really understand it – and she didn't
know the half of it.

With my newly emancipated life blooming, I was suddenly
pulled back on to the right side of the tracks when I met my future
husband at a family wedding. I'd been dreading going to yet
another function, but Mum was adamant that we were going out
in force as a family and that I needed to look my best. I'd never
seen this man before – implausibly our paths hadn't crossed. He
was an architect with socialist values, wore glasses and had a
geekiness to him, and I thought he seemed interesting and had
a nice face. He talked that night about so many different things,
perhaps for too long. Then I went back to London and forgot

about him. Until one day at Laban, somebody said, 'There's a postcard for you on the noticeboard. It's a Modigliani.' I turned the card over and it was from him saying, 'I found you.' As we'd told everyone I was doing art administration at Goldsmiths' College, it was quite something that he'd managed to track me down.

His family and my family were very much part of the same community and we both shared a lot of the hopes of our families. He'd lost his dad young and his mum was a widow living in Salford, while he worked in London. He began courting me by the book – we had no sexual relationship at all, which took me by surprise as this restraint was totally absent from most twenty-something men. After my experience with my previous boyfriend at university, I was determined not to be hurt again, so my barriers were up and unfortunately for 'us' he ultimately never became my be-all and end-all.

But he seemed like a good match and there was a lot of extra pressure on us because we were both members of a small community, our mums were both widows and there had been talk in Manchester. Shobna 'had been seen with him'. 'They are going around together in London.' Marriage very quickly became the only respectable thing for us to do. It would have been all right if I had been going out with someone outside of the community, but we were both Indian and everyone knew us and where we were from. There wasn't any grand proposal or romantic gesture; he didn't give me a ring. He just said, 'Maybe we should get married?' And I said, 'All right.' Our marriage didn't become a love story like my mum and dad's.

Strangely, my mum never seemed enamoured of him or our relationship. On the eve of the wedding when I was about to get my *mehndi* done, Mum disappeared to another party. It just happened to clash, and she knew I'd understand. It ended up being just me and the *mehndi* lady. I couldn't work out if it was just because she didn't care or if it was something else. It was probably not personal, but nothing about the wedding felt that special.

'**Oh, Shobna's getting married now, OK.**' She did what was right to support that. She was my mum and that was her duty. And she would do that to the absolute best of her ability.

Almost immediately after the wedding, it became clear that we'd made a terrible mistake and that things weren't going to work out. The truth is, we just weren't compatible and we wanted different things. I didn't even seem to be his type and we very rarely had sex – he didn't seem attracted to me at all. I ended up meeting several of his exes and they were all posh, gorgeous white girls, the kind of girls I could never be like, even if I'd wanted to be. Looking back, our hands were tied. I think he married me because I was Indian, I married him because he was Indian, and we both thought that was the way forward. On the surface, a true marriage of convenience. But I had been wanting a deeper relationship, with shared values and thoughts, whereas he seemed to be looking for something much more academic, something on the surface and I found that untenable.

His mother was another issue. We moved in with her for a few months after the marriage, while I travelled down to work in London four days a week, and she then joined us on our honeymoon. When we moved out, to a house just down the road, he told me she cried whenever she saw him and would say that I'd taken him away from her. He'd been living in London, so I didn't really understand what she meant, but I suppose it was because he was now living with another woman that wasn't her. Balancing the two of us was something he struggled with and it caused him more and more unhappiness.

We tried to save the marriage with a move to Paris, but by this point we'd both been unfaithful. Those weeks and months were very hard. We struggled financially and just couldn't connect with each other. To escape what was happening in my new Parisian home, I got into the contemporary dance scene in the Marais neighbourhood. I tried to build my life there and got some modelling and dancing jobs. But things at home became competitive, combative and antagonistic; we just couldn't see eye to eye. The final straw came when I was back in London on a job, staying with one of my old university friends, in her spare room, and he told me that he wanted to explore other possibilities and be with other people. I was so enraged – as I'd been completely honest about my sexual history and where I stood, and I felt very passionately that he should have told me that he needed time to explore things before getting into a marriage.

I basically drove back to Paris, packed as many of my things in the boot of my Volkswagen Mark One (a present from Mum) as I could, tethered the rest to the roof rack and left him. Mum was in India with my brother at the time, Sushma was living with her Danish husband in Singapore and Hema was with her South Indian family in Hyderabad, so there wasn't anyone I could turn to. I couldn't even explain it to myself, let alone to my family. I couldn't phone Mum and say, 'I've left my husband.' What would I have said? 'I have left my husband because we don't have sex and he doesn't fancy me, and I don't fancy him. And we've both been unfaithful.'

And so my money ran out and I lived in my car, back in London. I was desperately embarrassed and lost touch with friends, even though they had always supported me, because I couldn't face telling them what had happened and my weird new circumstances. I felt so ashamed that my plans had failed and worried that they would lose respect for me. I was desperately trying to work things out on my own.

Despite living in my car, I went back to working at The Place. While I was working on their 'Indian Summer Season of Dance', an actor I didn't really know well came to watch a show, and within minutes of speaking to me he'd suggested I move into his flat as he wanted to help me get my life back together. For some reason, it felt easier to open up to him than to friends who had been in my life a long time. I wanted to restart my story. I stayed in his one-bedroom flat in Deptford – he gave me his room and slept on the sofa and treated me like his little sister. He really saved my life.

As part of the 'getting back on my feet' project, I'd got a part in a play at the Theatre Royal, Stratford East. *Moti Roti, Puttli Chunni* (fat bread, thin veils) became an overnight sensation in London. I played a few roles and danced in the 'rain' on a moving set truck, in an affectionate homage to Bollywood. Though my parts were small, my costume changes were many. I had to change from being wet to dry in seconds, and I had to strip off at the side of the stage. The flyman said he didn't look, but he must have been able to see it all. One thing led to another and we fell head over heels for each other.

I never told my mum, nor any of my family, what had happened to my marriage, I hadn't been able to face anyone. Instead my ex-husband went around to Mum's to tell her. He said he couldn't offer me financial, emotional or physical support, and then he drove away.

She had said, **'Do you think I don't know my daughter?'** And she revealed to me that she had felt it wasn't right from the beginning and that I'd rushed into it. She told me that she felt a level of responsibility for the marriage because Dad wasn't there and she had known that I had been looking for someone to fill the hole he left. She said she should have stopped me, but the reality is I would never have taken her advice. It wasn't her mistake, it was mine.

And so, with these more open conversations taking place, I felt it was the right time to introduce her to my new boyfriend. I decided I wasn't going to hide my life from my family and that included him. She thought he was **'too quiet'**. Too quiet and too African-Caribbean, of course.

CHAPTER FOUR

Do you know I will always look after you?

A few months later my body began to feel strangely foreign and tender. I realized my period was late. In the tiny toilet in the Deptford flat, I did the test. A faint blue line appeared in front of me. And that was it. Terror poured into my life once more.

I couldn't work out how it had happened, as I'd been on the pill and we'd been using protection. While it had been a tumultuous relationship with lots of ups and downs, I did really love him and very much wanted to make it work. So, I told him I was pregnant with his child and he told me in anger that the baby wasn't his and that he didn't want to be involved with it or the pregnancy. He left me then, he left us. Me and my unborn child. I had become separated from my husband, single and pregnant with another man's baby out of wedlock, all in the space of a few months. The world caved in.

I didn't know where to turn or what to do. Eventually, out of desperation, I thought of my sister Sushma, who has always had a reputation for her practical, fair nature, but even she couldn't get over her dismay at what I had done. She told my mum before I had a chance to figure anything out, saying 'I didn't know how to help, but I knew Mum would.' But none of us really knew what the 'right thing to do' was, and my mother eventually came down to London to escort me to an abortion counselling session.

I will never forget seeing my mother's face when I met her off the train – it was complete disappointment. I felt her shame and horror so powerfully and I added it to my own. Despite her feelings on abortion, she had said she would support whatever choice I made. When we left the session, she turned to me and said, **'So do you want to have an abortion then?'** I said, 'No,' and she immediately replied, **'Thank God you said that, because I don't want you to either.'**

As we started to discuss what would happen, I felt closer to her than I'd ever been. We were finally in step with each other, walking the streets in London, her hand in mine, united by the unexpected circumstance and the shame following us and the family. In that moment, I felt her love would overwhelm everything.

'I will look after you in this. It is my duty to look after you.'

The sense of relief I experienced upon hearing those words goes beyond expression. Of course, it also stung because she said she would look after me out of *dharma* (duty) and not simply out of love, but that was her way.

And that was it. We had said everything we needed to. I waved her goodbye at the train station and she went back up north, while

I spent nearly my entire pregnancy in London. There was no space for me to be pregnant in Oldham and I needed to carry on working, so there was no question that I would go back with her at that time.

In London, I could be out and proud, celebrating my growing body in tight clothes, away from the prying eyes of the community up north. I grew more excited as the months went on, even though I didn't really know how much this baby would change my life. Occasionally I'd go up to Oldham because I was registered at both The Royal Oldham and Greenwich for my antenatal care. I'd spend the weekends hidden at home, or else keep myself very quiet in baggy clothes at family parties. When *Moti Roti, Puttli Chunni* toured to Manchester my mum's friends who came said that I'd put on weight, but that was not an unusual comment – at every social event I'd ever been to the auntijis were always talking about how much you had or hadn't eaten. It's a bit like British people and the weather. In the past, I'd always got stick for being too skinny. Now it was: 'You've put weight. Hasn't Shobna put weight?'

As a family we contained my secret because it was too shameful to admit. Raj and Hema were furious about the pregnancy and they felt I should be disowned. They were vocal about their feelings towards me and towards 'what I had done'. There was a time during the pregnancy when I got some worrying test results suggesting that there might be an abnormality, and Raj, now a newly qualified doctor, said I should consider a termination. In his eyes, I would not be able to cope with a different outcome. I didn't want to. I'd already had to consider abortion and was not going to go through that painful process all over again. I'd had this baby growing inside me for months, I'd become more and more attached to it as it had become more and more attached to me. I had a strong sense the baby would be what the baby would be. Despite the pressures of her other children, my mother defended me then and continued to defend my baby, who we had discovered would be a son.

The week before he came into the world, I was on the way back from a job teaching dance in London. I'd been stuck in the Blackwall Tunnel and suddenly I felt these strong bearing-down pains and I had no idea what to do. I finally made it out through the traffic and pulled over and can remember frantically looking in my car for anything that I could use. There was a bottle of water and some tissues, so I took them with me and squatted behind the car on the side of the road. What was I thinking? As if a bottle of water and some tissues would help me give birth. In that one moment I have never felt so alone. Seeing sense at last, I drove straight to Greenwich, and the nurses said that the baby could be born any day now. That scare made me realize I didn't want my son to be born in London, I didn't want to be alone. I really wanted my mum. So I drove up north.

Without knowing it, from that day on, I would never have my life in the south again.

My mum was there with me during my labour and was by this point an expert in the baby business. She'd not only given birth to her own four children but had been there for Hema's three and both of Sushma's. When we arrived at Oldham General, which of course Mum knew like the back of her hand, the doctors said I wasn't dilated enough yet, so off she went to visit some of her friends who were patients on different wards, leaving me sitting there on my own, totally petrified. That was Mum, she didn't mean it personally, she knew she'd be back in time...

I took gas and air – of course I was screaming for every drug under the sun, but that's all I got. I was completely out of it, cracking jokes every minute. I have some fuzzy memories of Mum shaking with her distinctive silent laughter at one point, who knows what I was saying, but I always could make her laugh. And I made the midwives laugh too. I remember asking her if she minded if I went down on all fours for the delivery – it's quite a thing, isn't it? To be in this position in front of your mum with your bum in the air, especially when we'd always been so covered up in front of each other.

And so Akshay, my son, was born. I cut his umbilical cord and whispered, 'You're on your own, kid,' with love, as he was free of me and my role as his host. Now that he was on the outside, he would be his own person and I would become his mother.

The shame didn't disappear after the birth. The lines I'd crossed ran so deep, like the permanent stretch marks across my belly, and I had this feeling that I had broken everything, not only within my own life but in my family's lives and the wider community as well. The culture of shame among North Indian Punjabi and wider South Asian communities meant that the dishonour I'd brought on myself for having a baby outside of marriage was shared by my whole family. It was a double whammy. The problem was that I wanted to live my life the way I did. I also didn't want to live like them, or perhaps I just didn't know how to live like them. I had, by all accounts, 'failed to do the right thing'.

It has obviously not been easy to 'live my truth'. Loving, being and living the way you want to comes with ups and downs. But for me to sleep at night, I've always felt like I had to do the best I could for myself. I did try and live the life they wanted for me – I had got married because I felt obliged to follow the path that had been set for me – but it just wasn't the way. Perhaps I was too young.

Perhaps I wasn't equipped with the necessary tools. Perhaps I couldn't ever accept the restrictive normative dimensions.

Perhaps I just wasn't them. I was the anomaly. I would always be the anomaly.

After the birth, we went home together, Mum, me and my baby. Mum fell instantly and totally in love with Akshay. It wasn't difficult, he was the cutest, most affable baby and he never, ever cried. She taught me everything. How to bathe him in the sink, how to feed him, how to soothe him to sleep. She made me feel so relaxed and she gave me so much confidence in it all. But it was very much her rules. When it came to weaning or potty training Akshay, I followed her ways for raising children with little argument. It was always her way or the highway, as I was beholden to her. I didn't have anywhere else to go, but I didn't want to go anywhere else. I was in awe of her expertise.

I only asked two things of Mum: firstly, that we never refer to Akshay's skin colour, in terms of comparing his darker skin to the 'blue' God Krishna. Every time I had met anybody in our community called Krishna or Krishan or Krishnan, they, more often than not, had a darker complexion. I did not want Akshay to be in that stereotype, however seemingly celebratory. Secondly, no one would sing the shame song whenever he was naked. I wanted him to feel proud of himself and not be besmirched with the shame of nudity and colourism that had haunted me all my life.

One day, Mum was going to a gathering with family friends and I decided it was time to face the music. I got myself together, with Akshay in my arms, to join her. As soon as we arrived, the questions started: 'Whose baby is this?' I can remember saying, 'He's my baby, Auntie,' about 20 times. This encounter sent the community gossip mill into overdrive and before nightfall I'm sure every Punjabi family in the country knew that Shobna Gulati had a dark-skinned baby that wasn't her husband's.

Now there was even more pressure on me to show that I could cope. I went back to work pretty much immediately. I was so emotionally dependent on my mum I was loath to be financially dependent as well, and I was determined to show everybody that I could support my choice. Mum took over most of the childcare; she became a second mother to Akshay. As close as she became to her new grandson, I didn't have a social life at all. It was an incredibly hard, lonely time. I filled all voids by working. I was ashamed, exhausted, unrehearsed and ill-equipped for parenthood and all the guilt I was carrying.

When Akshay was still a newborn, I landed a job in Leeds and the dates coincided with my cousin sister's wedding in India. I remember it was a week's dance residency and I would earn £500, which I desperately needed, so Mum took Akshay with her to be with the family before the wedding, and after my week of work I flew out to join them. The entire extended family was there and I definitely had a sense of foreboding about it and all the questions I'd have to answer, starting with, 'Whose baby is this?' It turned out that I was right to be worried – it was even worse than I'd feared.

Almost as soon as I arrived, everything exploded in my face. It really was as though a bomb went off, everyone arguing and shouting awful things about me. Pressurised by this shamed-filled gaze, Hema had said incredibly unkind things, things that you never forget, and there was Mum, caught in the middle, with her entire extended family watching to see how she would deal with it. She didn't stand up to support me, but then really how could she? In England she had shown me love in the purest form by supporting me in spite of herself and the disparaging looks and gossip from the community. But there in India, surrounded by her own family, she had no choice but to distance herself and my siblings from me. It was a barrage of blame, so I picked up my son, found a telephone and rang my Aunty Chitra, one of my dad's cousins, who I had confided in when I stayed in Delhi as a teenager. She became my rock again and put a roof over our heads for a couple of days before I managed to get a flight home.

When I got back, I applied for social housing. I had plans to move out with Akshay before Mum returned from India. There were so many thoughts and conflicting emotions in my head, but overriding them all was wanting things to be better for my mum. Me living with her had caused untold hurt and created a huge strain on the family dynamic. When we did finally discuss it, she agreed it might be better if I was living somewhere else.

Mum only ever visited the two-up, two-down we moved into once, to rescue me from a great spider invasion one night. I had been on my Amstrad PCW, printing out my CV as I thought it would be better for everyone if I became a teacher: regular hours, regular money, no more relying on my mum with my crazy work schedule. The printer was a daisywheel printer and it didn't just make a noise as it printed, it made my whole bedroom vibrate. At this disturbance something on the floor started to move. It was in the coir matting so I couldn't make out exactly what it was. As I bent down for a closer inspection, I saw at least seven large brown spiders crawling around the room. I'm a complete arachnophobe but I couldn't even scream because Akshay was fast asleep on my bed. It was about one o'clock in the morning, I didn't know who else to call, so I phoned Mum in a panic. She told me to put some glasses and cups over them and to wait for her. I was so relieved when, about a half hour later, she arrived and deftly threw each spider out of the window, one by one, using a small thin piece of

card she carefully slipped under the cups. She was my superhero
that night, but that was the only time she visited that home. (I
never lived that episode down and she absolutely loved telling
all her friends of how her 'independent' daughter was not so
much after all.) She continued to look after Akshay though, and I
regularly dropped him off and picked him up at her house, to fit in
with her and around my work.

Over the months that followed, she did try her best to
understand me, asking why I had chosen a Black boyfriend. I
remember once we were home watching *Ready Steady Cook* and
she leant over to me and said quietly, **'Him, do you fancy Ainsley
Harriot?'** Mum's experience of any Black people was extremely
limited to the few overseas doctors she'd met at the hospital – any
kind of understanding of their cultural background and history
had never featured in her life. I did appreciate that she was trying
to figure it out and confront her own prejudices.

Mum clocked everything that was going on around her. While
she may not have made a huge fuss, instances of casual racism
among her friends did not go unnoticed. Despite the pain and
disappointment, and her preference in some circumstances just
to rub along, she would challenge her companions. I recall a
particular instance involving a good friend and neighbour of the
family whose granddaughter had failed to secure a place at the
local sixth form college, while Mum's granddaughter had got
one. Her friend complained that there would be room for her
granddaughter if it were not for all of 'them Pakistans', followed
by the caveat that, 'I don't mean you, Asha'.

Mum had replied, **'What do you see when you look at me?'**

Even in that moment, Mum saw it as an opportunity to educate
her friend rather than simply be angry. She explained some of
the history of the British Empire in India and how, when the

British left in 1947, to add insult to injury, one of their parting shots had been to divide India. Mum was seven years old when this happened and her parents had already moved to Mumbai, but her family (her paternal uncle, aunt and two cousins) who had found themselves on the wrong side of that arbitrary border were brutally murdered in the mass exodus as they fled their home. Of their surviving children who had escaped the massacre, one of the girls came to live with Mum and her parents. This terrible history is a part of our lives.

As a family, like many others affected by Partition, we never talked openly about this atrocity – it was too much to bear. But in my attempt to share this chapter of our history, I did finally engage with the truth of what happened, through a TV programme called *Empire's Children*. This programme held the first-hand account of my late Aunty Shanti's horrific experiences on that day when, as a young girl, she witnessed the murders of her parents and brothers and hid under their dead bodies until the threat was over and she could escape to safety. Mum helped me to encourage the family to finally share their terrible ordeal, and it was no easy task to begin to uncover this truth.

So Mum, heavy with the weight of this history and the blatant ignorance of her friend who had known her for over 35 years, wearily said, 'You can't keep on dividing and ruling us. If you accept me, you have to accept us all.'

Through her example, Mum set the bar high. This is something I have always been able to hold on to when I had my own similar experiences of being disappointed with some of my white 'friends'.

Mum and Dad were different. Dad had embraced every community and as a GP he had been exposed to so many people from different backgrounds. The truth of it is that traditionally

Punjabi and North Indian communities can be really, really racist. Some believe colour can literally determine a person's worth. Ideas of people are based exclusively on skin, and 'fair is beautiful' no matter what. You've just got to look at the skin lightening or skin whitening ads in India for the grand scale of this paler skin aesthetic. Matrimonial ads feature phrases such as 'wheatish complexion', 'light' or 'fair-skinned' and these attributes are held up as the pinnacle of skin perfection.

Conversely, to be dark-skinned reveals that you're from the wrong side of the tracks, and ugly. Though not being directly brought up with those particular values by my parents in England, we were discouraged from spending too much time in the sun or making ourselves look 'too tanned'. I remember the horror expressed by my dad's older sister-in-law when I had visited Mumbai, after a couple of weeks of sunning myself on the beaches of Kerala as a young married woman. 'Thank God you're married, Shobna, and not single. You've become so black, it's a wonder your husband still wants you,' she said in disgust.

I do feel that, within our community in Britain, there should have been a deeper understanding of the non-white minority experience. Working in the performing arts meant I encountered people from so many different heritages and I embraced our commonalities as well as our differences. I found great empathy for the shared struggle and so my friendship group extended far and wide.

I had experienced racism throughout my life, both directly and indirectly. When I worked as an Indian dance teacher, I found myself in Minsthorpe, an ex-mining community in South Elmsall, Yorkshire. I was met with a diatribe from one particular parent: 'I'm not having my lad learn any Paki dancing, from a Paki woman.' I also experienced racism within my friendship group of

Indian heritage, indeed I was once sent an opening night card for a play I was in that pictured a black stallion; needless to say the play was not *Equus* or *Black Beauty*. I felt every slight acutely.

For some in my North Indian Punjabi community, their bigotry and prejudice were deeply rooted in their colourism. A kind of internalized racism hidden deep beneath their Brown skins, under the historical, structural and institutional layers of racism that were used to prop up the brutality of the British Empire and colonization, wherever it went in the world. Colonization throughout history, especially from western nations, has instilled a colour hierarchy with white at the top. And so, having emigrated to the UK, my community didn't want to be lumped into one homogenous non-white group. It filled them with fear and further fuelled their ignorance of the 'other'.

It is more prevalent in the older generation, but it also exists among my peers, especially in tightknit cultural groups. The human desire not to be at the 'bottom' of the hierarchy pile, combined with their experience of the colour standard, fed into their desire for social status to place them above those who were (mostly) darker-skinned – whereas 'white' people were definitely all right. Some of my childhood friends had married white people and this was seen as a step up – any other 'mixing' of heritage was not.

My mum did recognize racism and she fought some of the school battles with me when Akshay was regularly called up in front of the class for so-called wrongdoing, when white children were not even penalized for doing exactly the same thing. He would often be in detention for hair styles that were just a part of his culture. She went beyond her own life experiences to try and bridge the knowledge gaps that my son's father had brought into her life. She didn't shout about it – instead, her understanding of herself and of people evolved.

There were so many issues, beyond just those of the
community with its supposed 'racial' boundaries, which I'd
crossed by having a child of dual heritage, and in helping me
to raise my boy, she tried to make sense of all of that. She'd say,
'We are one human race, Shobna,' and it wasn't just words, she
truly believed it. Indeed, I don't think there was anyone she loved
more in the whole world than Akshay. In her eyes, her family had
become just like the Benetton campaign, championing diversity
and representation in a time when nobody else was doing it. We
were ahead of the rest and were moving with morality rather than
against it. She held her head firmly above that parapet and decided
that she was no longer taking any prisoners. She began to be proud
rather than ashamed of what her family had come to represent.

Over the years there were people who were interested in
marrying Mum, but she wasn't interested in any kind of romance
for herself. In strict Hindu communities, widows can't remarry.
My father had been so liberal, though, and nobody actually said
she couldn't have made that choice. But for Mum there was never
any question that she would ever move on, whether that was
down to latent cultural attitudes or simply because of the depths
of her feelings for my dad. Mum spent more of her life as a widow
than as a married woman, but it was her role as my father's wife
that she would always identify with. She saw herself as a mother,
a grandmother, and a widow to my dad, and in her eyes they
remained an enduring love story.

There's no doubt that she was definitely lonely at times, and
the squirrelling away of things to make her feel safe and secure
reflected that. But her house was rarely empty. Raja didn't leave
home until he was 30, when he got married, and then Akshay
brought fresh energy into her life. Hema's children would all also
live with her at certain points while they finished their education

back in the UK, so her grandkids kept her busy. She also travelled everywhere with Akshay. They went to see her old school friends in America, they went to India together for more family weddings (but this time without me to ruin everything). With Aki, duty became love. But with me, duty remained duty. I'd upset the applecart and I was a girl. I couldn't have expected her to forgive me.

The kind of work I was having to take on, and just working in the arts generally, was punishing while also raising a kid, but because we were always broke I could never say no. I made the decision to apply to do a teacher training qualification, which would mean I could become a language teacher. I thought if I managed to gain some independence from my family and slot into a regular routine, where I didn't have to rely on my mum, it would be better for us all. Up until then, I would be away working on a play, choreographing or teaching in another part of the country for a week or two and Mum would have Akshay, till the weekend, when I'd be back. She'd take him to nursery when he was older and do all the things I should have been doing during the weeks I was away. Then I'd be home, and he'd be with me again. I felt hugely grateful to Mum for everything she did for us, but I also felt deeply indebted. I did feel that my brother and sisters were constantly judging me for leaning on Mum, even though she would say she missed Akshay when he wasn't with her. But I wanted to provide a steady life for us all, to try and take some of the pressure off Mum and the 'shame' off me.

Just before Akshay's third birthday, I got a call from Victoria Wood's team for a new sitcom, called *dinnerladies*, that they were putting together. My agent called the same day as the audition to say I'd got it. I ended up missing the train back, but when I finally made it on, I called Mum to say, 'I think our lives are going to change completely'. She said, '**I do hope so, my love.**' And just like that, life did change almost overnight.

This would be the first time in my career to date that I would be working on television as a performer. Not only that, but with my comedy idol, Victoria Wood, and the BBC. If you don't normally see yourself represented in a space, you think that it's not available to you. It works at a subconscious level. All the letter writing to production companies and auditions for TV that had been unsuccessful had left me seriously doubting whether I would be able to further my career. That's also why I had applied to become a language teacher. Theatre roles were niche. Yes, we were creating our own work and I was dancing, teaching, writing and choreographing, but we were never recognized as 'mainstream'. Or indeed, celebrated by 'the mainstream'. Best to keep us in that little box (you know, the ones we tick on theatre equal opportunity forms, for their diversity reckoning, not necessarily for our advancement or further representation).

I was beyond thrilled at getting the *dinnerladies* job. It just so happened that Judy Hayfield, the casting director of *Coronation Street*, had met me some months before, for an audition to play Mike Baldwin's 'fancy woman'. I hadn't been successful in that instance because, despite my real age of 31, I looked too young (you see, Brown don't frown). But Judy had said she wouldn't forget me and she kept her word. Unbeknownst to me, Victoria had been asking around at Granada for a girl with a playing age of 23 plus, of my heritage with a soft Lancashire accent, and Judy put me top of that list. When I finally met with Vic, well, we got on 'reet good'. I'm going to call her Vic, because that's how she introduced herself to me from day one of filming, while she made me a brew.

My audition was in the basement of the old Granada studios, by the breeze block walls and pipes. Seeing her sitting there, just like it was an everyday occurrence, was surreal. She seemed shy but quite stoical, and she immediately made herself relatable. There was something about her that I recognized in myself. Something that I do too, to push pass my feeling awkward. She 'dryly' perused my CV looking for TV credits, found none, and commented on my very academic background, which she found amusing. Then I had us all laughing as I admitted that, from her beautifully constructed script which I'd been sent in preparation, I didn't initially know what a lilo was. So I switched round the script to reflect my ignorance in order to find the truth of the Anita character I was playing (where the joke is that Anita didn't know what a dildo was). Anyway I got the job, because Vic said she would really enjoy making me, this very clever woman, dim.

I was working alongside ingenius, famous, funny women with prestigious track records. The show was an extraordinary challenge for me, and it was a real first in TV comedy. Outside of the safe bubble of female comedy standup, sketches and duos, this was a sitcom based on the lives of a predominantly female cast: dinnerladies not dinnergentlemen.

It did change my life. I was late to that big break, in my thirties, and since then, I have been afforded many opportunities, some of which I have run with, though at times the label of 'nice but dim Anita' has been hard to shake. (Sometimes, I think casting directors do not recognize you can be an actor, because you have Brown skin.) Vic always fought my corner if work came up and I was right for it, and I really miss her voice, even though her genius lives on.

To say Mum was a soap fan is probably the understatement of the century. She was obsessed with them, they were a part of her every day. Sometimes she would have two TVs on at the same time, so she didn't miss anything. She watched them all: *Emmerdale, Coronation Street, Eastenders,* daytime soaps, night-time soaps, midday soaps, soaps from the south, soaps from the north, soaps from Australia. But *Coronation Street* was always her favourite. When she'd first arrived in Oldham, they had rented a television and Dad had asked her to watch *Coronation Street* to help her understand what the north was like. He wanted her to learn the local dialect and understand the sense of humour and way of life. This was back when *Coronation Street* had just started – it was only six or seven months old. She was a young mum and had come from a fairly posh family, where they spoke proper fancy English. '**The Queen's English,**' she would say. She was, after all, a child of the British Empire, where it had been a requirement to learn it. Well, Oldham was different, and my dad thought she needed to know how northern people talked and behaved in order to better acclimatize.

From that moment on, she watched every episode of *Coronation Street* and that's how she learnt how people spoke and the anecdotes, and the bathos and pathos style of comedy which came hand in hand with being a northerner. She came to appreciate the slightly comic passive aggression and the nuances of northern culture, and she saw the bittersweet life of the people who lived here. 'Aren't you doing well, Asha, for someone who's come all the way from India? Oooh, you are good at English, aren't you?' By this stage in her life she knew precisely what they meant.

In 2001, after the second series of *dinnerladies* ended, I landed a role in *Coronation Street* and I was able to move out of social housing. That marked a transformative moment in my relationship with Mum. And not just because she was such a mega fan and she lived for the *Street*. The story pretty quickly went from everybody talking about me in such a bad way because of my failed marriage and 'dark-skinned' baby born out of wedlock, to Mum saying, **'Well they're all calling me now, because you're on television, aren't they?'** with a wry smile. She knew exactly what was going on. She'd been bathing in my shame for so many years that it was life-changing for her to now be able to bask in pride. Obviously, it wasn't ever as though all was forgiven, but it was definitely a positive addition to our previously fraught relationship. *Coronation Street* also meant that I was able to raise Akshay in one place. The guilt of not being there for him had been overwhelming, the guilt and the shame of relying so much on my mum – all of that started to go.

Mum and I still argued, especially when it came to my relationships. I'd been caught up in a very destructive and abusive situation with a man I'd met while I was pregnant with Akshay, but after close to ten years I finally got myself away, and I eventually spoke to Mum about it. I told her everything. Sitting facing each other at my childhood kitchen table, where I had never been able to eat my breakfast, she knew that there was something wrong, that there had been something terribly wrong with me for years. So she asked me and I told her the truth.

Even though I'd had other 'public' boyfriends during that time, this man was always there in the background, always ready with cruel words or physical threats, whatever harm he wanted to inflict on me. When I finally confessed what had been going on, my mum was very shocked, but she shared a secret with me too. She told me something about her life, something terrible that had happened to her as a child and that nobody had believed her about. She told me because she had seen a reflection of her experience in mine, but we never revisited it. I kept Mum's secret – I didn't share it. And she kept mine. We never spoke of either again, we'd said what had been said, and we just carried on being mother and daughter.

But there was a shift in our relationship and we had definitely come to a new level of understanding. The shared memories we gave to one another, hidden from the world out of shame and fear of exposure, rejection or being disowned, planted something in our relationship that continued to grow for the rest of our years together. We learnt that no matter how big, burdensome or taboo our secrets were, we could trust each the other to hold them and not judge one another, and instead support and foster resilient strength from them. These memories, these stories, this period, destroyed our existing relationship in order for us to rebuild it upon surer, stronger and more honest foundations. The shame of abuse, of being a woman, of telling the truth, of having desires, of breaking boundaries that had been decided by long-dead ancestors who had made us keep things hidden from the world and each other – this became our stronghold.

The only thing I couldn't shake was how my choices had affected my mum, and I always wished that there could be a way I could repay my debt for her support of me at my lowest, weakest and most unacceptable. She found a place for both me and my son. Her love became more powerful than my shame.

CHAPTER FIVE

Who are you calling a racy lady?

Asha Gulati was a control freak.

I don't mean this as an insult, but in order to understand my mother you need to know that she had a complete and utter need to manage everyone and everything, however large or small. This meant that whenever she sensed her control and power ebbing in a situation, she would develop some kind of reaction to defend it. Sometimes that would be a straightforward argument, but often it would manifest itself in other ways, such as the bags and bags of stuff and piles and piles of papers she accumulated for the years after she lost her husband and therefore her place as a married woman within the community. These mountains she built between her and the world around her began to rise higher and higher, ever edging upwards towards the ceiling, and claimed more and more physical space between her and the world. They formed a barricade behind which she felt safe and secure. My siblings and I would try and break through these ever-growing walls in pleading tones:

'Let's put this stuff in boxes and organize it all?'

'Perhaps if we throw some of it out it would help you work out what to keep? At least, we'd be able to see the wood for the trees...literally.'

In her own matchless way, she forcefully rebuffed each and every attempt. Of course, her hoarding was meticulous and methodical. Envelopes were relieved of their plastic windows and gummy strips, so the paper recycling wouldn't be contaminated by the plastic or gum. All used stamps were cut out with a 3mm border and collected for charity. The newspapers had the adverts neatly snipped out and recycled, leaving only the main body of the pages. There was order and process to these mechanisms, and she closely policed whether we too had correctly recycled our envelopes. These stringent rules, her fastidious attention in deciding what she could be rid of and what was essential, made her feel more in control of the chaos that her life had descended into after the death of my dad.

I wonder if I subconsciously decided not to pay attention to the signs? Or were they not clearly defined enough for me to risk her wrath by addressing why things just didn't feel quite right? My mum was vociferously independent, and she was instinctively insular in many ways. Indeed, I would go so far as to describe her as the most self-sufficient person I've ever known. She'd had to become so extremely able after she lost her husband – she'd had to find a method of keeping the family together. Ever since, she had always occupied her own private space, desiring little input from anyone to keep herself busy and her spirits level. She needed so little of the world or those around her, to the extent that in her company you could feel entirely surplus to requirements.

She would sit in (at least) two M&S cardigans. Mum, like all her friends, always loved the aspirational clothing label, St Michael, the quintessential 'English' brand (though it was in fact founded by Polish refugee, Michael Marks, in 1884). She would wear them over her loose-fitting clothes and sit on the edge of her bed, with her back against the radiator, grumbling as she looked through the window at a cloudy grey sky, and say, **'The only thing hot about this country is the mustard.'** Surrounding her were unfinished crosswords, neatly cut out of the paper, her specs and *Roget's Thesaurus* not far from reach. Her island, that she and she alone inhabited, was her power source and we children had acclimatized to this apartness.

Like a papyrologist, Mum gloried in her crosswords and paper archives and none was more extensive or exhaustive than her collection of my press cuttings. From when I was a young dancer and had appeared in the local rags, she had cut out and kept every single clipping about me. As my career took off, the volume increased and people across the community would send her cuttings of anything they'd seen – some of it good and some not so good – and she stockpiled it all as if she were the record keeper of my life. The information collation and ordering of Shobna Gulati's story became a task that she undertook with an almost professional devotion.

The strangest part was that she squirrelled it all away. I had no idea of how large this red-top library had become because she rarely mentioned any of it, nor commented on anything that was written about me. The exception was when someone attacked me

– that's when she sprang to my defence. I remember she was sent a cutting of a theatre show I'd been in, right at the very start of my professional career. It was a picture of me in *Moti Roti, Puttli Chunni*, dancing in the rain, my costume clinging to my curves, with a little note accompanying the cut-out making it clear that the sender disapproved. I can still picture my mum's wry smile, knowing my shyness concerning my body. **'Darling, if you've got it flaunt it,'** she had said. She wasn't willing for anyone outside of our family to make any judgement calls on me. That wasn't their place. *She* was the record keeper and it was up to her what was acceptable.

The first and last time Mum let slip about her quiet yet all-consuming undertaking was when I finally made it onto the covers of all of the TV guides and soap listings. That had been a real battle – these magazines had never had a 'South Asian woman', or actually any woman of colour, as the headline picture on their covers before. As major storyline after storyline had been relegated to subheadings, I'd put my foot down with the *Coronation Street* press office and said that I wouldn't be giving any more interviews until they put me, Keith Duffy and Jimmi Harkishin (who both played the love interests of my character, Sunita) on the cover.

When I finally made it onto the front cover, much to my surprise, my mother confided in me that she'd gone to Asda for her weekly shop and had been so excited she'd had to rush back home to collect her Instamatic. She'd returned immediately to take a picture of the rows of shelves with me on all the covers of the magazines. It was so unprecedented, and as a closet feminist, Mum wanted to capture and celebrate the first time culturally representative TV and soap magazine covers appeared on the supermarket shelves. It was a victory on all sorts of levels. I had been at the forefront of this cultural revolution in

TV magazine front covers. I was astounded at her revelation – I could hardly believe she had been so excited about something to do with me.

In the early noughties, *Coronation Street* was *the* biggest thing – we were sometimes getting audiences of over 15 million – and as one of the stars I became instant tabloid fodder. It wasn't like today when there's streaming and so much choice of what to watch. Back then, we were in people's front rooms nearly every night at the same time, and the level of intimacy that people developed with you was incredibly intense, which led to them wanting to know everything about you.

The only press story that ever seemed to matter was my terrible offscreen love life. Journalists had discovered that I'd had Akshay outside marriage. According to their headlines, I had kept that part of my life hidden and the tabloids were overjoyed to uncover this skeleton in my closet. I was now *famously* – or infamously – a shamed woman, and the whole thing became chip wrap fodder. The papers tracked down my ex-husband, photographed him, and then extensively quoted 'a source close to the family' who said a lot of not-so-pleasant things about me. These articles emphasized that I'd been married when I became pregnant by another (mystery) man, which was true, but neglected to mention that I'd been very unmistakably separated from my husband at that point.

After reading the headline about my so-called 'secret wedding' to my first husband, my mum folded it up, **'to come back to later,'** and said, **'Well, I don't know why you're so upset, you look quite good in that photo.'** She was leaning against the radiator in the front room, a pile of papers in front of her, and took off her glasses to reveal that her imitable smile had also found its way into her eyes. It was the day after England had won the Rugby World Cup and my picture was alongside a photograph of Jonny Wilkinson holding the Webb Ellis Cup. **'It's not all bad, Shobna. He might notice you'** – she pointed at Jonny – **'it could be worse.'**

Once again, Mum was forced into fielding the calls from the 'concerned' community of extended aunties. 'Shobna got married in secret and you didn't invite us, Asha?' they would say. After my mum explained that the only wedding I'd ever had was to my ex-husband, which they had attended, there'd be a brief pause from the aunties before they said, 'Oh, that one,' and the phone went dead.

Every other week there seemed to be another story about me, stories which I just couldn't work out how journalists had managed to get their hands on. I was dating another soapstar, who was in *Emmerdale*, for four years. We would be followed, photographed and constantly speculated about. When that relationship ended any male friend or acquaintance I had would be open to conjecture.

Later on in my stint on *Coronation Street* I was dating a well-known Manchester DJ. The papers seemed to find out everything about us, places we went, what we did and our arguments – not just that we had them but specific details only the two of us could have known. It didn't make any sense.

Obviously, a lot had happened in my life, and there were a lot of things I hadn't worked through properly. That had an impact on some of my behaviour and it would have been hard for me to hold down a relationship in any context. But with these stories continually coming out and things which I would have very much liked to keep private from my family, let alone the whole country, becoming public knowledge, I lost it. I didn't trust my boyfriends or my friends. And they didn't trust me, as I accused them of selling stories about me and they accused me of leaking our personal life out into the world. It was only years later that I realized my phone had been hacked by the Trinity Mirror Group. No one had betrayed me, the journalists were simply listening to my voice messages and injecting my own words into their column inches for so-called 'public interest'.

My mental health was in tatters. I was also worried about what it was all doing to my young son. In a small town, my increasingly sullied 'reputation' was gaining momentum and we were the furnace fodder for the rumour mill. After a long week on set, I'd dread the end of Friday afternoon phone call from the *Coronation Street* press office as the team would let members of the cast know if the Sunday papers were carrying a story about any of us. If you couldn't completely deny an article, the papers would run it regardless of any additional fabrication or exaggeration. That's what sells papers, after all. I would then have sleepless nights worrying about the headlines, the taglines, what my mum might see, what my young son might think, what my family, friends or the community would say...Everybody would extrapolate something.

If I'd had *that* call, I would wake up before the crack of dawn on a Sunday and rush in my car to Manchester Victoria station to look at the batches of the papers, just so I could prepare myself by reading the headlines. That was the only power afforded to me: knowing what people would know and think about me later that day.

But throughout all this, Mum didn't bat an eyelid. She wouldn't blink at racy pictures where I'd be showing off my lacy knickers or wearing lingerie, nor would the lewd headlines cause her much bother. **'More mirch to the masala,'** she'd say: more chilli in the spice mix. And all the while, she was surreptitiously cutting out, piling up and hoarding these sordid stories and pictures, to keep track of what she couldn't control. Sometimes she would make my sister Sushma buy an extra copy of a magazine or paper if she'd missed anything on me.

If I was embarrassed by my own behaviour, I'd try and conceal stories from Mum and the rest of the family. I was by no means perfect and sometimes didn't make the best publicity choices for myself. Regardless of the content, Mum collected it all. There I was stashed away with numerous articles and photographs of the Queen, Audrey Hepburn, David Beckham, Posh Spice and their growing family, and Lady Di too, who was still getting press coverage years after her death. Mum loved them all, **'kindred spirits'** she called them, **'except that Camilla'**.

Mum's desire to keep a vice-like grip on the reins of my life sometimes undermined our relationship, though of course now I've considered how much of it was innate to her personality and how much was a foreshadowing of her already faltering mind. One of the most hurtful things she'd do was show me up in front of the wider family. There was one holiday in Canada, another family wedding, which my now teenage son, my mum and I attended. Everything was, **'What does she know?'** I'm not sure if she did it to make it clear publicly that she was still punishing me for my transgressions or if it was just that she resented me, but it was incredibly awkward and obviously hit a raw nerve for me.

I wondered if she wanted to remind me that she was the matriarch, to assert her dominance and control over me as my success became more established. We could never just be two women as equals – she would always be my mother first and foremost. I was now in my mid-forties and had a dynamic career in my own right, so it was hard for her to reconcile that with the old Shobna who had disgraced her family. After these kinds of outbursts I would go and find a quiet space and cry. It would be the sting of shame from years ago, but also the shame and hurt afresh as it came out of my mother's mouth.

At the end of 2011, Mum and I went on a trip to India. I had the opportunity to properly spoil her because I had a little bit of spare cash since I'd been working consistently and was in between good jobs. So it was just the two of us, sometimes sharing a bed as we stayed with family. We had some great moments on that trip. Flying into Mumbai, as the announcement to refasten our seatbelts on the landing approach came across the tannoy, Mum was so excited she began singing, **'Aye dil hai mushkil, jeena yahan, zara hat ke, zara bach ke, yeh hai Bombay meri jaan'**, which loosely translates as 'Oh my heart, life is an uphill struggle, be alert, be aware, this is Bombay my love'. Then she impersonated the actor from the 1956 film, *C.I.D.*, **'Aha ha ho hoo hee hee aa hmm hmm'**, shaking her head in true Bollywood heroine style, then collapsing into a fit of silent giggles at her out-of-tune singing. With a huge smile on her face as she peered out of the little airplane window at the hazy 'city of dreams', she was overjoyed to return to the place where she had grown up and fallen in love.

On another leg of our trip, in Gurgaon, I remember really making her laugh with jokes under the *razai* (a traditional quilted blanket) about my sometimes unkempt appearance. Mum was very fond of having 'perfect hair', with not a strand out of place, so she would wear an old salwar kameez in bed. Wearing this outfit also meant there was no bare skin for mosquitos to bite and it kept her cosy if the air conditioning was on. We'd laugh and take pictures of her having wrapped her head in the *dupatta* (scarf) to keep her hair 'flat'. At breakfast the same scarf would be used to 'hide her modesty', ever elegant and gracious.

But there were absolutely horrendous moments too. Lots of them centred on making plans. Mum would have to offer her point of view on every part of our itinerary. If I dared to chip in, she would say, **'What has she got to say about it?'** as if I was going to put a spanner in the works of whatever we were planning or talking about. It felt as if she'd almost forgotten that I'd grown up and that we had moved past that kind of dynamic in our relationship.

One night I had gone out for a late-night coffee in Mumbai with my cousin sister-in-law, just for us to escape the flat and catch up with some 'girl time' away from our parents. We came back just before midnight to complete Armageddon. Mum was pacing up and down, my uncle (my dad's brother) pacing the other way. Frowns all round. **'All this time drinking coffee, eh? Why go out for coffee shoffie when you can make it at home?'** They had been worried sick that we could have been caught up in some religious celebrations that might have turned sour. I kept thinking, But I'm nearly 50…and very streetwise!

One evening on that same trip, I glimpsed a burn on Mum's back. It was very rare for me to see her in her vest top, or really to see any of her bare skin. If we hadn't been sharing a room, I would never have seen it. I asked how she got it and she said that she'd been sitting in front of the radiator trying to get warm and hadn't noticed it burning. That really worried me. I thought, How caught up do you have to be with what's on the TV, to be sitting there and have the radiator burn your back like that? But everything else seemed completely as it always had been and I just presumed it was a one-off. We didn't dwell on it, we both just put it down to being 'one of those things', and I simply put some cream on it to help her skin heal.

I came away from that trip with the overriding feeling that nearly all the progress we'd made over those years with our relationship had suddenly taken a nosedive. It was as if we'd stepped back in time and the anger and resentment that she felt towards me a decade before was all back in full force. It was as though the intervening years had never happened, as though they had been obliterated from her memory. What could I say? Choices I'd made had huge consequences for my mum's life, and I couldn't change that.

These confrontations really tipped over when we got back home. One evening I took Mum out with me to a restaurant opening: Asha's, owned by Bollywood singing legend – and Mum's namesake – Asha Bhosle. The living legend herself was going to be there, so I'd taken Mum to get her hair and nails done, something I always adored doing with her. We had a fantastic meal and she'd just loved all of it. She'd had photographs and an autograph. The plan was I was going to drop her off at home and then come back into town to meet up with some of my friends at a jazz bar. By this point Mum's mobility had been in decline and the jazz bar had lots of steps down, so it wasn't practical for her to come with me. It wasn't in any way an unusual plan or something that Mum would have ever questioned. But from out of nowhere, she went absolutely mad. She was as angry as I'd ever known her and she clung on to that rage for weeks after. She wouldn't speak to me on the phone, she didn't want to see me. She wouldn't tell me what I'd done wrong. I was inconsolable.

Her anger reminded me that, from the moment I was born, she had seemed cross with me for not being what she had hoped for. I had learnt to bear this. But this time it seemed so extreme and uncalled for. I wracked my brain – what could I have possibly done to upset her so much? Was it because I was having a good time? Was she angry that I went to meet my friends? My siblings said to me, 'What have you done this time?' and I didn't know what to tell them. In their eyes it was nothing out of the ordinary because of my past disagreements with Mum. But as her reaction was so hostile, and because we'd seemingly been having such a lovely time, it kept me spinning.

Here we were back to India again.

Back to when I became pregnant.

Back to being a divorcee.

Back to being an outcast.

Back to when I was a kid.

Back to being Little Miss Controversy.

Back to all the terrible times I thought we had overcome.

And I suddenly thought, Does she just hate me? Has she hated me from the minute I existed?

Did she still resent me for not being a boy, or for getting on with Dad? Is it more than just because I had a baby with a man who wasn't my husband?

I couldn't find the answers, and my thoughts were wild. I internalized all of her behaviour and interrogated my memories to try and understand the exact moment that had turned her against me.

I was transported to places in my own memory I had forgotten, back to a time when I was a child and Mum and Dad were adamant that I needed to see 'someone' because there was something 'wrong' with me – I was too 'unusual'; I didn't conform. The help came in the form of a child psychology specialist, one of our 'uncles'. (I remember I had found it strange that Uncle was a specialist in children but didn't have any of his own. Woe betide me if I shared that opinion though.) Mum and Dad had discussed their 'third child syndrome' theory and then sent me to speak to him.

His conclusion: 'Shobna misses attention from her parents, her dad in particular – this gives her a psychosomatic tummy ache' (although when I was an adult I was diagnosed with coeliac disease, and suddenly it all made sense). 'This makes her act out. She's obviously been displaced by her brother and this is her way of vocalizing it to you.' I didn't know if this were true, all I knew was my tummy hurt and sometimes I would find it difficult to eat. I would hide or store food and then I would be reprimanded by Mum for not eating.

Her anger was so visceral after that night at the restaurant. I remember so clearly believing that my mum didn't like the person I was – and that wasn't something I just imagined, it was something she said to me often. I thought of her lack of praise for anything I'd achieved, even when it was something that pleased her, and the ways she would always compare me unfavourably to other girls, whether it was at swimming or dancing, or just among girls in my community. My body, my nose, my face, my discipline, my grades, my behaviour. It was all a let-down to her.

Out of the woodwork of my earliest memories came narratives I had purposefully forgotten. My mum telling me that I didn't deserve to have nice things because I couldn't be trusted. I didn't keep things the way she wanted me to. I was the idiot, the owl's daughter, who was irresponsible, scatterbrained, unkempt and couldn't care less. If my homework came back with a bad mark, it was because I was thoughtless. If I didn't swim well in my lessons, it was because I wasn't paying attention. If I had misplaced my Tupperware, or even my repurposed ice-cream container 'lunchbox', I was too careless. It's as if she kept a record, a list of black marks against me, every indiscretion and slip-up that proved time and time again how I had disappointed her as a daughter. When you contrasted my experiences with my brother's, whose very breath warranted applause, it felt as though she had very little real affection for me.

Another flashback came to me, of Mum explaining that my

uncle had checked my horoscope in India and found that I was destined to be unlucky. It's as if my mum's holistic disappointment in me had been drilled so deeply into my consciousness that it had become part of my DNA. It couldn't change. I had been oblivious to how enmeshed it was in our relationship, but this new anger was not 'new' at all, it was an old lifelong anger that my mother had always had towards me. It would never disappear and it could never be resolved or absolved. It had been following our relationship around like an ever-looming shadow since I came into this world.

I too had fallen into the past to try and make sense of my mum.

From the autumn of 2009 onwards, although we visited Mum at home, nobody really ever stayed overnight, or spent any extended time with her. All her children and grandchildren had flown the nest, and there was nobody keeping a watchful eye, which meant Mum was more able to keep her secrets and conceal quite a lot from us. The only exception was when she had been in poor physical health. Mum had experienced a heart attack in her mid-forties, before my dad had died, then had later been diagnosed with a congestive heart condition. In 2003 she had heart bypass surgery, and then in 2014 she was diagnosed with bowel cancer.

For some time before her cancer diagnosis, Mum knew there was something wrong, but didn't let on to us. She was getting the blood in her stools, but her GP just asked if she had piles. Mum said she hadn't, despite having had four children. We had all noticed she'd become a little thinner, but none of us put it down to anything out of the ordinary, with only herself to cook for now. Anyway, we had been told it was better for her to carry less weight, as that meant less stress on her heart.

Frustrated by her GP's response, Mum sent a sample off for

more evaluation. Further tests revealed she had a tumour in her colon. It was a devastating diagnosis. After all the heart surgery, now this, and things were to get even worse. One night she was due to come to the Royal Exchange Theatre in Manchester with my brother to see me in a series of short plays. Instead, I got a distressed call from Raj, stuck in a traffic jam on the M60 motorway. Mum had called him to tell him something was seriously wrong with a pain that started in her leg.

Raj thankfully got to her just in time. Mum had done all she could to manage her situation, including using one of my son's old stripy blue and yellow football socks to compress her leg. My brother diagnosed her immediately with thrombosis. Due to a change in her medication leading up to her surgery, a blood clot had developed. He rushed her into A&E and then called me to say not to worry, she was comfortable, and to finish my work and come to the hospital – by then they would be ready for surgery.

I did the play in a whirl of emotion. Work has always been my safe place, my place to go to in trauma. I don't know how I got through it as there was nowhere to hide in this very wordy two-hander play. As soon as I finished, I drove to Oldham Hospital.

Up until that moment, my brother and I hadn't really been speaking. We'd had a big falling out and my mother had had to intervene. The fact that my mother initially blamed me entirely, added insult to injury. We were on polite but not intimate terms. But at this moment we were together by Mum's bedside, with no real knowledge of where the blood clot might have travelled in her body. Mum seemed very chirpy, making jokes about how frugality could even help beat away mortal peril. **'*Beta*, you never know when an old pair of football socks can come in handy,'** she laughed. I helped the nurses scrape off the last of her glamorous gel polish manicure, my heart racing all the while. She said she had wanted to wait to go into theatre, so that she could see me. I just said, 'I'll see you again in a few hours, Mum.' I didn't say goodbye.

After they wheeled her away, I turned to Raj and said I would be there for him. He was so capable as a doctor, yet so distressed as a son, and I felt compassion as a sister for a brother. After, I called my sisters to reassure them. Somewhere inside I felt Mum wasn't ready to go, but whatever was going to happen, I would be there for everyone. I was so unusually calm. I was spent, maybe I had used up all my adrenalin during the performance earlier in the evening.

Minutes turned to hours and hours to still more. Eventually, we found out that the surgery had been successful, and the clot was no longer life threatening. A few days later, Mum was back home. But it was by no means over.

Then we began the next journey together: the one with cancer.

Over the next few months, Sushma, Raj and I took it in turns to take Mum to radiotherapy. Seeing this tall, fine-figured woman become more diminutive by the day was gut-wrenching. She was tired and fed up with everything that was happening, but she was still Mum, finding a twinkle in her eye for her radiotherapist, who happened to be a handsome young man.

The experience shattered us all. I was in between jobs, but Sushma and Raj were fitting appointments around their everyday lives, family and work. Bearing witness to her deterioration, her fatigue from the radiotherapy and her lack of appetite felt like a stab to the heart. What we failed to pay attention to at all were the vivid stories from Mum's past which suddenly began to resurface. Some of the stories were nostalgic and charming, others focused on terrible trauma she'd buried for decades. We didn't see them as dots that could possibly join up; her mental depletion was obviously a result of her body's problems, not her mind's.

It took Mum a very long time to recover from two surgeries within a few months of each other, and she was totally exhausted. Friends visited her in hospital, but she wasn't particularly lucid and the radio was on constantly in her room. Because she didn't want to eat hospital food, I began bringing in her favourite food in a bid to try and make it all better. She wanted her comfort dish: Punjabi kadhi and rice. We affectionately called it 'yellow curry' as it was flavoured with the healing spice of turmeric, creating a rich, deep golden colour. Kadhi and chawal, a sour soothing combination of healing spice, salt, natural yoghurt and gram flour tempered with mustard seeds and curry leaves. That magic formula soon did the trick and she slowly began to regain her appetite. She was coming home.

Mum had weathered so many physical storms that it became second nature to explain away momentary slips in memory or unusual behaviour. The doctors had even cautioned us that her treatment for cancer and the trauma of surgery could lead to disorientation, so obviously that's what we chalked it up to. Post-surgery, Mum needed 24-hour care at home. Luckily, I had little work on, so I was there. (Unluckily, the expectation that I was always going to be there began to rear its head too. For some of my siblings, my work was often misunderstood as a 'bit of fun'.)

Eventually, to everyone's relief, Mum was declared clear of all signs and symptoms of cancer. Her physical health remained steady and that it had ever been a major concern faded from our minds, perhaps because we wanted and needed to see her as strong and capable. She had brilliantly adapted to the stoma, something so out of her comfort zone, that she'd been left with after her bowel cancer operation, and that really reassured us all. Her plan was to get herself strong so they could reverse the stoma and get back to her normal. She once again found the determination that had carried us through so much and returned to her role as the family backbone.

Looking back, I think she had already started to ask me for help, I just hadn't been able to decipher her messages. Whenever I went over to her house, I'd always bring food with me because she wasn't exactly fond of anyone cooking in her kitchen. Mum always supervised, which was about the most stressful thing you could imagine. All you had to do was start chopping an onion and she was on high alert. It was like she'd be sitting in the other room just waiting to hear a bowl chink or the cutlery clang. She'd shout, **'What fell? What's broken? What are you doing? Be careful!'** She had, of course, her certain ways of loading the dishwasher or using the cooker, and she always said that we broke things or messed things up whenever we dared cook there. Even the oven was sensitive to her touch. So I decided that I'd make food at home and avoid the battleground of fighting with her over her kitchen.

But one night she quietly said to me at the front door, **'It's silly you making food for you, me making it over here, we should share our food.'** I didn't really think about the fact of her allowing me to prepare food in her kitchen – didn't notice that her pedantic nature and ownership of her kitchen had vanished. I couldn't really fathom that she might actually want me to help her. Or indeed, that she was asking for help in her own cryptic way. I go over and over that in my mind even now.

I did, however, start to notice that Mum's driving was becoming erratic. To be honest it had never been exactly stellar. The car had always been a bit like a therapist's couch, where Mum took on the role of the therapist and you became the patient. She'd put you on the spot and ask you things she wouldn't bring up anywhere else, then she'd dole out the advice which she expected to be followed. Part of me loved it when we drove together, because there was a sense of straightforwardness you didn't get from her at other times, but part of me would dread clicking my seatbelt on, because you just didn't know what home truths were going to be served up to you as the car's pistons fired.

Now, for a few months, it seemed that she was driving faster than usual. We made it into a family joke, Mum getting a bit of a reputation as a silver speedster. That year she got a birthday card saying 'Racy Lady' because she'd picked up so many speeding tickets. But then she also started to lose her way in streets that were so familiar to her.

In 2015, Mum was ill again, with a respiratory infection, and had lost a significant amount of weight. We worked out that she hadn't really been eating properly for a long time. She was so habitual in her ways that she'd have her breakfast, but then seemed to forget about food unless someone was coming over to see her. She was still doing the food shopping and bringing the same old things back from supermarkets that she'd always bought, but they were just left sitting in the fridge uncooked. She would eat a bit of toast and jam here and there, but she wasn't really cooking, making vegetables or rotis from scratch, or taking in any proper proteins. A few months after she recovered from cancer we slowly started to refer to Mum's 'situation' as it became more opaque. A rain cloud that had been dodging us and that we hoped would be blown away seemed now to be getting closer and darker each day. The contents of it would change the course of our lives.

My brother Raja, the doctor, suspected something wasn't right, and said that she should go for some tests. She threw the mother of all of mother's fits at Raja's gentle suggestion, but in the end she complied and aced them all, scoring highly across her maths, times tables and dates. I remember we laughed over it, thinking that Raja had overreacted in that way that all doctors probably do when it comes to their jobs, never mind their mums. She would say, **'I'm not gaga, he's just like his father'** (in being so overly concerned without cause).

But then new loose threads began to unravel in front of us. Shifts in our mother that were hard to explain away. Shifts that demonstrated a lack of certain traits that had been central to our mother's character. That was the first time that anyone mentioned anything to do with her losing things.

Asha Gulati had always, always been very, very careful of her possessions. Objects and artefacts were extremely important to her. She always said that she and Dad struggled hard to get the things they had, so if you lost anything it was seen as something terrible, as a stain on the sacrifices and struggles they had undergone for the benefit of all. In her view, if you lost something, it was entirely your fault and you deserved to suffer for the loss. Once, as a kid, I lost an umbrella. I was done for. It was a beautiful thing, a pretty vintage brolly that Mum had loved, and I'd left it on the bus. The sense of dread at telling her crushed my chest because I knew what was coming. It wouldn't be the normal level of disappointment and hurt – instead I knew it would play deeply into the narrative that my mum wheeled out whenever I did anything wrong, the **'Shobna is careless'** story. I knew it would be difficult to borrow anything ever again.

So one day, it must have been in the autumn of 2016, when I was over at hers looking for a pen to write her a note, I opened a drawer and found a neatly folded sliver of paper with a faint outline of her handwriting in pencil on both sides. I unfolded it to find a little note written to St Anthony, the patron saint of lost things, asking if he would please, please help her to recover a pair of gold hooped earrings and a necklace.

Please St Anthony you have helped me in the past. Please I need to find my walis and purple amethyst necklace. Please help me. Thank you so much for your help, Asha.

And then on the other side of the paper:

A miracle. (Plus a list of more things she'd misplaced).
Thank you St Anthony for my walis, keys, earrings and necklace.

Of course, she hadn't mentioned that she had misplaced anything of value to any of us. In later months, as I spent more time in the house, I discovered notes tucked away everywhere – in little tins, in among her sewing stuff and oddments, in the corners of her cardigan pockets. It became apparent she'd been losing things for a long time and had been trying to silently bargain with St Anthony for their recovery in Bombay-style 'Blingish'. St Anthony would be fluent as he had been so much a part of her Catholic education in Mumbai.

Mum's possession of her possessions seemed to be loosening and she couldn't trace how they came to be missing. She was constantly getting held up whenever she got ready to go out. If I came to pick her up, we'd find ourselves spending hours searching for the back of an earring that she had wanted to wear. Sushma would have the same story on any visit up from the south – she would spend her time helping Mum cleaning and emptying the hoover, looking for the ill-fated back of that earring. The ownership and control she had spent all her life rigidly holding onto began to scatter like dead skin. It gradually became clear that she had spent a long time trying to find and reinstate the missing, cut-out pieces of her memory, which had become like her Swiss cheese newspapers, piled up around her house – no longer intelligible to anyone else but her, as they were filled with too many mysteriously cut-out gaps.

At the beginning, the lapses had seemed trivial and like 'normal' things that happen as your age ascends, so we didn't pry behind the curtains she wanted to keep drawn. And why would we even think to? She had been so dominant, instrumental and powerful in our lives, and we had learnt only to ask what she allowed. This did not allow or permit us to point out or examine these new weaknesses. Why wound her pride and question her independence? Equally, we were afraid of what would happen if we began to expose what she was concealing, as we knew deep down that it would be the end of so much of what we had fought hard to protect.

The thing is, she was often still herself, full of jokes and her usual dry wit. She'd still make sure that everything was her way or the highway – no middle ground was to be found. She had become grumpy about everything though, and when I say everything, she was grumpy even at Christmas. At every Christmas. But then, she had a history of being cross – that was just the way she was – so nobody noticed her impatience worsening. We just thought she was turning into an even grumpier older woman. At family parties and gatherings at home, we'd put her irritability down to all of us being there the whole time, invading her space. It was because the kids were all too noisy, getting in the way of her soaps, or she was raging because we'd used her kitchen and broken something. There were constant explanations.

Mum had grown used to her own company and she liked her house to herself. But what became impossible not to notice was how tightly she was hanging on to the things that upset her, especially towards me – such as the night of the restaurant opening. She wouldn't bury things and move on, she would cling on with a steely grip so tight it began to become unmanageable.

For months this went on. None of us could predict the trajectory or the timeline of how the situation would play out. These days were frightening for all of us because she had always been the one guiding our family ship. And now suddenly she wasn't.

It's hard to be completely sure, but I believe that she did have an idea that her mind was failing her. She started becoming selective and secretive about what she told us. She put memory hiccups down to other things like her bowel cancer, her heart condition, or issues with her stoma causing her brain to cloud. Mum was comfortable blaming physical things, as they were 'real' and tangible to her. But she refused to acknowledge out loud, even for a second, that she could be struggling mentally.

Slowly, piece by piece, the image we had of my mother began to look less and less complete, as though someone was gradually dismantling a jigsaw. The pieces by themselves didn't feel significant, but as a collective they began to reveal a very different person.

Asha Gulati was very frugal. She had always had a specific way of brewing tea, with a strict ratio of two bags to three cups. You would have to warm the teapot first, swill hot water round, empty, then fill again with rolling, boiling water up to the top hole (God forbid if you underpoured). After the tea was brewed, she removed the tea bags after squeezing out every last drop, and piled them up by the sink, later cutting them open and spreading the tea leaves in the garden as compost and to keep the cats away. Thriftiness made up the very texture of her being.

When it came to cooking with anything that came in a tin, like peeled plum tomatoes or soup, Mum forced us to wash the tin out with water to make sure every last scrap was accounted for, then you'd have to put that liquid into the pan to make sure that every last drop was used. Mum's curries were always that bit runny, but she could never be accused of wastefulness. And when it came to eating, every morsel had to be scraped or soaked up until your empty plate resembled hers. To our children 'Nani clean' was the greatest accolade.

Outside of the kitchen, the philosophy was the same. Come Christmas time, she brought out sheets and sheets of flat ironed wrapping paper (she was a passionate ironer) recycled from the year before and her baskets of ribbons that she'd been saving since January. You had to open your presents very, very carefully and peel off the Sellotape gingerly because she'd be mad if you snagged it. Cards would all be put to one side and then cut around any writing inside to make gift tags for the following year. Any string or wool would be repurposed and, because she was so good at sewing, old fabric would turn into a patchwork quilt for refugees or a patch-up for threadbare clothes. Nothing, absolutely nothing, went to waste.

One day I saw my mum put a tea bag straight into a cold cup – what we would call mug tea – and it felt, in that instant, as though my heart was being pierced. I could just hear her voice saying over and over again,

'Two tea bags in the warmed pot, fill the water up to the top hole.'

'Two tea bags in the warmed pot, fill the water up to the top hole.'
'Two tea bags in the warmed pot, fill the water up to the top hole.'
'Two tea bags in the warmed pot, fill the water up to the top hole.'
'Two tea bags in the warmed pot, fill the water up to the top hole.'
'Two tea bags in the warmed pot, fill the water up to the top hole.'
'Two tea bags in the warmed pot, fill the water up to the top hole.'
'Two tea bags in the warmed pot, fill the water up to the top hole.'

Mum had never drunk mug tea in her life. It was wasteful. Back in the day, she even sometimes made you carry the teapot through to her sitting room to show her that you'd followed the instructions. But there it was, she was making herself tea in a mug.

Other practices started to fall away, but it sometimes took weeks before we realized. No one with memory loss ever lets you know they have forgotten something so automatic and instinctual, because they can't remember having done it in the first place.

More and more of her began to go missing.

Asha Gulati was always right. If you didn't like her opinions, in general, that meant you were wrong. It was never that you could have a difference in viewpoint. And we all listened. Every sentence would start with **'No, but.'**

It was while I was listening to her espouse her opinion on something, holding court as usual, that I noticed that whenever new people would enter the room she'd repeat the same stories to them once, twice, even three times. It seemed almost comical. Initially I thought maybe she was doing it as a joke. But she kept on talking about the same things again and again and didn't seem to register that she'd said it before. She'd say, **'You don't listen!'** One day, I nipped out for a breather from the tension at home and Mum phoned me seconds after I'd closed the door behind me. I realized that it wasn't the first time – she had begun to telephone me often to ask me little things, things she should have known the answers to.

The sand was shifting beneath all our feet, but I remember in that instance feeling like it was only me who'd registered another commonplace, everyday irregularity. After all, I was always on hand so it wasn't a surprise that I'd be the one picking up the first signs.

More random pieces of the puzzle started to disappear, my mum was becoming an ever more abstract figure. It was so incremental and inconsistent. Some of Mum's habitual actions disappeared but then returned with a vengeance a couple of weeks later. She'd suddenly be there, at your shoulder, watching how you were making the tea. Similarly, months could pass without us noticing a new addition to the pile of lost pieces.

I'd stayed with Mum after her cancer diagnosis and recovery, then in 2015 to early 2016, I toured internationally in *Mamma Mia!* – which meant I was away for longer periods, once up to six weeks in South Africa. While I was away, Mum ended up picking up a dreadful respiratory infection. It had made her so ill that she was hospitalized. When I got back, I started staying with her to make sure she was eating properly and help build her back up.

I didn't realize it at the time, but my new career, of becoming a carer for Asha Gulati, had begun.

Her driving problems escalated. One day I cried throughout a whole half-hour journey with Mum because she was driving so quickly. I thought we were going to die – crash and die or else kill somebody else. My God, she was so cross with me when I told her how scared I was, even though I tried to rationalize with her and explain that the police would stop her from driving, if she drove like that. **'Get out of the bloody car if you don't like it, stupid. I'll be the one driving. Dafa ho** [get lost]. **Jao** [go]. **Dafa ho, jao!'**

These explosions were followed by uncharacteristic warmth. Not long after that terrifying drive, I drove her car to pick up some material for something she was sewing and accidentally clipped the back of it. I expected her to admonish me, but instead she said, **'Never mind, darling *beta*, it happens to everyone.'** She then regaled me with stories of when she had first learnt to drive and how she'd got all sorts of bangs and knocks secretly fixed without Dad knowing.

It felt disorientating.

After that day, we started driving her everywhere. Instead of getting into standoffs that would last for days, we started to try to protect her without confronting the issue in hand. We'd say, 'Oh Mum, you don't need to bother to drive, I'll come with you...I need something from there too.' We had to ensure it felt like Mum's idea, because she would then feel in control and that would prevent her from losing her temper. However, after a run-in about driving with my son, we disconnected the battery of her car.

Yet many days offered moments when the veil was lifted and I could see right through the steamed-up glass exterior of her life. The closer I pressed my face up to the cleared glass, the more I was able to see everything within. Confusion and fear ruled.

The day of the manic car journey, I got home and immediately started googling all of Mum's symptoms. I typed into the blank white space as many words to describe the combative and erratic behaviour she had begun to exhibit as I could think of.

Old people and erratic driving.

Old people and moodiness.

Combative behaviour.

What's wrong with my old mum?

Why do old people get violent?

Is it normal?

What are the symptoms of someone being senile?

Repetition of the same story.

The stories of her childhood she shared over and over again. The moments of tenderness suddenly cancelled out by sheer force of the anger. Her irrational grudges and terrifying driving. It had stopped being something I could sidestep.

The search results were pretty conclusive. Mum was displaying classic signs of mental deterioration, namely dementia.

CHAPTER SIX

Do you think I am mad?

Memory is like a filing cabinet of oddities – arbitrary details of our sensual experiences stuffed into drawers that jam, chance calendar dates we have to rummage through every year. There is a hierarchy here at play, with some of the more important and emotional folders kept within easy access, but this doesn't mean that the anecdotal or seemingly insignificant events aren't logged and stored away too. And many of our files are a mixture of pleasure and pain.

Mum returned home to her childhood time and time again, sometimes finding joy but also experiencing an acute pain in her nostalgia. She was all grown up now. What are we without our memory? When we cannot access our imagination or personal history, or find our foundations in those fundamental pillars, do we stop being human? Do we become then a condition and no longer a person?

Our ability to sequentially organize the folders in our mind and make them available at a second's notice is something we don't even realize we have. It's like the air we breathe; we expect information to be there because it always has been. But as I began to care for my mum, I gained a new perspective on memory and the organization of time, and my own perception of how it operates and functions change. Mum's clock didn't keep ticking round in an orderly dependable fashion, it began to jump around and strike at random. No pattern, no order, just moving of its own accord. Sometimes frantically and at other times imperceptibly slowly.

Mum's aptitude for remembering everyone's birthdays was a perennial superpower, but by the end of her life she couldn't remember how old any of us were or indeed, how old she was. Sushma was pleased that she had knocked a good 20 years off her last birthday...even if it meant being 20 pounds short in her present (Mum always put the cash in our cards, saving all the new notes and shiny pound coins religiously in preparation for the birthday giveaways). But without an internal system, chronology disappeared, for there was nothing to tether it to. Days collided, years slipped away and events from decades before were brought into the present. I felt like Chuck Noland in *Cast Away* – I never knew what the tide was going to bring and when Mum, like Wilson in the movie, would cease to be.

We have an understanding of time as an inalienable progression from past to present to future. We can't even conceive that it could possibly operate in any other direction. But in other traditions this linear view of time isn't so deeply embedded. The Mayans and Ancient Greeks had their own ideas of recurrent time; Buddhists and Hindus base their karmic beliefs on what goes around comes around. Hinduism teaches us that time is cyclical, the *samsara*, with each age proceeding in a merry-go-round as we walk the wheel of time between birth, life and extinction. Nirvana is billed as freedom from that eternal cycle, a place where we can finally find peace. But some of us lack the cultural context to appreciate that time, or our memory of it, can be reasonably experienced in any other way than through the 24-hour clock. It was just December, so now it's January. Our lives are supposed to be a sequenced experience which keeps the steady rhythm of a ticking clock, and that's how we organize them.

But caring for my mum offered me a view of a different structure of time, one in which the journey is uneven and repetitious, and in which the tide of memories stop taking their cues from the calendar and instead present themselves at random.

Sitting in front of the telly, listening to Mum talk, I always used to think about the looms of her memory weaving and I would begin to examine the loose threads discarded along the way. A new picture began to emerge. Mum was unlocking areas of her life she had once sealed off to even those closest to her, and from the chaos came another history.

In the very earliest years, before the diagnosis, when we had just a tiny niggle that something might be up, she'd be midway through a conversation and then suddenly started talking about some story from when she was a new mum. The conversation became disjointed, but not entirely out of character – your parents are always going on about how lucky you are in comparison to how hard they had it, and they're always using their stories to drive this message home. But when Mum's initial signs of animosity and forgetfulness came into focus, so too did a new relationship with the present. The only constant was her, so in order to stabilize disorder she placed herself at the epicentre of the whirlwind of her memory. As an outsider, I can only describe it as seeing someone get sealed off from the world and locked into their memories, as if they have fallen into themselves. She was living in a dream which was actually once reality, and one out of which she couldn't be shaken. She didn't want to wake up from it.

Mum was no longer the woman I knew her to be. There were the constant confrontations over her medication, erratic driving, stories repeatedly caught on the loom, the fridge full of the week's groceries that she had wanted but that remained uneaten. And there were the things that simply went missing, both belongings and truths. She had always been an incredibly sincere person with an unshakable moral code, but she'd begun to play fast and loose with the facts of what was happening to her.

It wasn't just her pride or obsession with control that was at the root of this new secrecy. It was more her absolute horror at a new word that had started to be whispered, firstly by my brother, but then by other doctors too. Culturally and linguistically there was a lot that was muddled for Mum – and for many people of older generations – around the language of mental health and decline. Becoming more senile was totally acceptable and seen as part and parcel of the aging process. Everyone would eventually become a little absent-minded and doddery, that was just the circle of life, and she would often joke about how she was forgetting stories and people's names, **'like an old lady'**. She didn't joke about forgetting to eat though. Or the sheer amount of misplaced items she could never find. To Mum, her state was natural, not diagnosable. And when it came to probing more into her unusual behaviour, she would completely shut down. Curtains drawn. Door shut. Head back into an old newspaper.

It was my brother who first raised the alarm in a more medical way. As a doctor and the son of a doctor, it's in his very DNA to want to solve and restore people's lives to normalcy and good health. So to diagnose 'what was wrong' with our mum was at the forefront of his mind. I think he felt responsible too, as he was her son and the man of the family, and she had always relied on him since my father died. My sisters and I looked to his lead when it came to 'the situation', but none of us wanted to pin down what was actually wrong, or say it out loud. What I noticed day to day I often didn't pass on.

Actually, I wasn't brave enough to give my opinion. And at the end of the day Mum would only really take medical advice from my brother. He was the professional, and he had that professional courage. Yet despite being firmly the apple of my mother's eye, she was furious with him:

'My son thinks I'm mad.'

'I am not losing my mind.'

'He's telling all of you.'

'You all think I'm going ga ga.'

Mum was right, she wasn't mad. And she never would be. But her mind was suffering an accretion of losses every day.

From 2015, as a family, we had started to discuss the possibility that Mum's behaviour wasn't just a by-product of her physical conditions. It started light-heartedly, with the little observations and quizzical looks, but fairly soon we were sharing more unsmiling concerns with one another, collating it all together into a more definitive and focused direction. By the end of the year, we couldn't escape it – whether you were hearing the same story for the seventh time or watching her drink loads of tea made in her big mug – the cracks widened and we couldn't not worry what structural damage they were reacting to and buckling under.

However, as far as her doctors were concerned, there was no cause for concern. Raj had made sure that Mum underwent a raft of tests designed to establish what we were dealing with. They discussed the possibility that she might be having mini strokes or even a bad reaction to some of her medication that would knock her out of kilter. Of course, in the back of our minds there were thoughts that it could be something else too, but as Mum was so reluctant to confront it we found it hard to form the words, even privately.

For years Mum had been stoically keeping the side up through countless health and family crises. When she lost her husband at 45, there was a lot of talk of her mental state, as there often is with widows left behind. Words like manic, anxious and frantic would be bandied about. 'Asha must be hysterical,' was the constant whisper from family and the wider community. I can so distinctly remember the doctors around my mum after the news about Dad had so shockingly arrived, each trying to tranquillize and subdue her.

In the aftermath, it was of utmost importance to my mum that everyone saw how stable she was, how firmly in control of the whole situation she remained. There could be no chinks in her mental armour. Later, Mum had to contend with the shame associated with me, her daughter who had disgraced the family name. Because she, as a mother, had chosen not to disown me and had instead personally helped to raise my illegitimate child, she became a pariah by association and her judgement and mental state once again came into question. Perhaps there was a sense that her decision wasn't the sane one. Of course, such ambiguity only made her even more zealous in her attempts to assert her command over the situation. Throughout her life, Mum had fought to keep herself out of the 'unstable' bracket and everything she valued in herself and others – capability, self-control, discipline and presentability – were all wrapped up in that battle.

Dementia was entirely incompatible with my mother's worldview and her place in it.

As an English, Punjabi and Hindi speaker, 'dementia' translated into her mother-tongue simply meant that she was demented. Wild, irrational, unkempt, frenzied. Simply put: mad. The loaded words which describe dementia across the languages she understood also seemed to exacerbate Mum's repulsion. Dementia to Mum meant a total and utter loss of control, which was the antithesis of every facet of her identity. Even the most tangential mention of her possible condition incited the full Asha Gulati volcano to erupt.

This, of course, was wrapped up in the conditioning she had experienced through her family and community. Any kind of mental decline, outside of 'regular' old age, is a massive taboo in South Asian communities, where mental health struggles of nearly every shade are often brushed under the carpet and kept quiet within families. Dementia is a physical disease, but even in our community today there is such a stigma surrounding it that for those who suffer themselves or care for someone with it, diagnosis can be incredibly difficult. Dementia isn't seen as a disease or a physical syndrome which causes mental deterioration, it is seen as a mental defect and something to be ashamed of.

For us, 2016 was a really difficult year, mostly because our suspicions were time and time again dismissed. Raj tenaciously continued to put Mum in front of doctors, but every time there was a test Mum would pass with flying colours. There is no one experience of dementia. In fact, there are as many versions of dementia as there are minds that suffer from it. There is a wide range of symptoms and it evades a clear trajectory or prognosis, which often makes it very difficult to diagnose.

In Mum's case, it was more about the small clues we pieced together. One of the hints was in the way she would doggedly cling on to any family 'slights' and arguments from the past, not just the ones involving me. My niece, Mum's first grandchild, Hema's eldest, had got married in a quiet wedding ceremony, very much immediate family only, so it hadn't involved Mum. She was so *so* cross when she was told. Sushma and I had to deal with the fallout for weeks afterwards. I didn't have an explanation for the secret marriage – it had come as an intense shock to me that my niece didn't invite Mum to her wedding day too, but Mum took things to the next level and would not let it go. She felt totally snubbed as she had been there for her granddaughter, always.

Going through it with Mum over and over again was tiring, and I felt resentful that it was left for me to sort out. It felt like another drama on top of everything else, and the *everything else* was hard enough. The aggression around her tablet taking, for example, had reached fever pitch. We had daily rows over whether or not she had taken her doses of medication, the problem being that Mum would often forget what she had and hadn't done. It made us very anxious, as we knew these tablets were keeping the deterioration of her physical health in check – without the right doses it would lead to more health issues which she could ill afford. Mum would insist that I checked all the details with the pharmacist, because what would I know about her tablets? She would say, **'What do you know? You are not a doctor. I know what to take, they're my tablets,'** so I would have to text my brother to ring her and reassure her, because she would listen to him. We were all on edge and it was becoming difficult to manage.

Mum continued to phone me often, pretty much immediately if something had come up in her head. She couldn't wait to have her question answered, she needed it sorting there and then. I was beginning to feel very overwhelmed. One day I nipped to my own home to pick up something. The second I arrived, Mum phoned, so I left my house in a whirl, perhaps not securely shutting the downstairs window. Within ten minutes I got a call from my neighbours saying that they had tried to apprehend thieves in my house. Dashing to and from Mum's house became my modus operandi and it was panic-inducing.

I turned 50 that summer of 2016, and my mum was very much a part of the celebrations with the whole family. I held three family events, and at the tea party with all my friends who knew her Mum was in her element. Witty and funny and glamorous, Mum was the life and soul of the party. She was proud and happy to be eating lovely cakes and bijou sandwiches while drinking prosecco and copious amounts of tea. But I caught her looking at the balloons with a faraway look and childlike joy. She was there some of the time, but at others I could tell her mind was elsewhere, steeped in her own past.

My niece eventually had a party to celebrate her wedding in November 2016 (thank God), so all was forgotten and just about forgiven. But midway through the celebration, Mum had fallen dangerously ill, with her recurring respiratory infection. She was hospitalized and we were again thrown into a spin. Luckily over that period my sister, Hema, was visiting from India and Sushma was also in Oldham, so they were able to settle Mum.

It wasn't until January 2017, when she had an MRI scan that showed small, historical strokes, that Mum was officially diagnosed with a mixed dementia, including vascular dementia. My brother and niece (who is also a doctor) explained that Mum had chronic infarcts (cerebral infarctions are areas of dead brain tissue resulting from a blockage or narrowing of arteries) in parts of the brain related to the functions of spatial awareness, language and thought processing, and in the part of the brain that relays information to the cerebellum (balance, walking, coordination and so on). The scan showed that there was no evidence of extensive dementia changes and that Mum's memory problems were due to old strokes where small clots had stopped the blood supply to parts of her brain, depriving them of oxygen, or in medical terminology, ischemia. It was this process that had led to vascular dementia, by which Mum appeared to have been mildly affected at this point, though her doctors said her condition wasn't too unusual.

Just before Mum's birthday, Sushma brought her and Hema down to Leicester to see me in a production of *Grease* at the Curve Theatre. It was an eventful trip, as it always was, because you had to keep a keen eye on Mum. The family who had taken me in when Dad died were now based in Leicester, and I was staying with them, so Mum was able to get a good comfortable break on the journey and catch up with old friends. At the end of the week Mum celebrated her 77th birthday with my three siblings and my son, but I couldn't be there as I was now in rehearsals for *Anita and Me* in Birmingham. At points in the tour, I could commute back and forth to care for Mum, but when I couldn't the family WhatsApp chat was filled with increasingly fraught discussions over the new dosette box (pill box) and how difficult it was to manage with Mum's care schedule.

Mum had always used small brown medicine bottles to separate her various tablets. Everything became even more confusing for her when the dosette box was introduced, but it was the only way we could properly oversee her correct medication. Raj was tasked with reorganizing the medicines and we drew up a care plan for while I was away working. I would be the weekend carer, depending on my work and performance schedule, Sushma

would do Monday, Tuesday and Wednesday, Raj would cover
Wednesday evening into Thursday and Akshay would come up
from the south to be there Thursdays and Fridays. We all had our
roles.

Sushma really came into her own during the times I was
working and would spruce and clean the house from top to
bottom and ensure all the shopping and cooking was done. Raj
would check on her health and look after paperwork, while
Akshay would hang out and make her favourite masala beans on
toast (Heinz beans, made with fried onion and a pinch of garam
masala, and topped with melted cheese). He'd also walk to buy
her favourite snacks from Greggs or the chip shop. I would shop
and cook when I could, but I was also often so exhausted from
performing and travelling that I'd just enjoy sitting in her living
room: listening to her stories; organizing hair, nails and eyebrow
grooming, to keep Mum looking neat and feeling herself; and, of
course, watching television. We all watched TV with her and that
became her portal into life outside of her own. We watched the
same programmes over and over again. Even now, as I write this
during the Covid-19 lockdown, Sushma and I watch the Channel 5
weekday afternoon films and reminisce at the welcome break they
provided from all the ITV murder mystery repeats.

So, even though the official diagnosis was in, she still
managed to score 70 per cent in the reasoning tests designed
to help identify dementia. Blood pressure issues are a common
cause of the vascular variant of dementia, which was something
that Mum had struggled with since the heart attack in her
forties. Her kind of dementia can affect your reasoning,
planning, judgement and memory. It can come on immediately
after a stroke, or it can, like Alzheimer's, progress slowly over the
course of many years.

It seems the cruellest thing, that the tiniest little clot can starve your brain's blood vessels for one night while you're sleeping and fleece you of your most precious memories. And that is what had been happening for months, if not years, to my mum. It is entirely incurable; the only question is how fast it will progress.

While we were all obviously crushed to have our worst suspicions confirmed, it was also a watershed moment in terms of us being able to explain to ourselves what we had been going through. But for Mum, even after the diagnosis, which was as black and white as the cut-out newspapers piling up in her house, nothing changed. She point-blank refused to accept it.

I wasn't working as much in March and April 2017, so I spent nearly every day with Mum, giving Sushma and Raj a well-earned Easter holiday with their families. We installed cameras in the hallway by the door and in the kitchen to keep an eye on her safety and security when we physically couldn't be there, but mostly I was able to stay and it was Mum and me together.

During this time, it wouldn't be quite accurate to say the present didn't exist for her. It was more that it began to operate only as a prompt for the cogs to turn and release another moment from her history that had been locked away in the filing cabinet of her mind, as though she had just stumbled upon the key for another locked drawer. It was certainly true to say that she was starting to live in her own realm, which was only adjacent to the one the rest of us were in.

In some drawers lay secrets never shared, of losses and estrangements, but sometimes the outside world would trigger memories that would enrage her because they brought back trauma she had deliberately buried. She had been estranged from her youngest sibling for decades, after he'd got married within a period of mourning for their father. Mum saw that as disrespectful, and to make matters worse, the wedding went ahead before their mother was able to come to the UK. She often went back to that difficult time during this period.

We'd be watching something on TV with a tea and biscuit in hand and suddenly something said by a character sent her back down the rabbit hole of time and she'd emerge mid-row with her brother. '**I don't know why he's gone,**' she'd say. '**I don't know where he is. Why has he done this?**' She'd rake through their conflicts over and over again. Sometimes the story itself would disappear and she would just experience the emotions surrounding the loss of her brother. Sometimes she would be confused and ask where he was now, as if it had happened that morning and she was experiencing it for the very first time. She could become very distressed and disorientated, as though she was constantly travelling between different planes of consciousness.

Over time the memories she went to became more concentrated, and she returned time and time again to her childhood. Considering that my dad had been the anchor of her life, and even after she had lost him she had so firmly and consistently identified herself through the role of being his wife, she lost him from her memories very early on in her illness. He just ceased to exist for her, except peripherally. Occasionally, we would be back to the time when we were teenagers and Mum was wrangling the four of us to school, Mum treating us like the children she thought we were, but even then Dad was never really mentioned. The man who had meant so much to her became a phantom in her memories. He just slipped out. Decades of life with him, her best friend, her only love, were stolen without her notice.

In the mornings now Mum always slept late. She had increasingly become a night owl and a very grumpy morning person. At 8am, when I poured my first cup of tea, I'd smile and think what a total role reversal it was: Mum still in bed, sleeping late like a teenager, while there was me at the kettle, ready to make the brews, having had a sleepless night worrying about her. I'd often get up in the dark of night and go in and check on her, concerned that her stoma bag was on properly or else to turn down the volume of the ever-constant TV. (In some ways she could be very sharp – a dementia diagnosis doesn't suddenly mean you become slow-witted. Mum had worked out that we'd put the TV on a timer and was adept at turning this off, so the box would be on all night long. *She* was the commander of the remote control.) Mum regularly referred to me as a *sariboothi* (Punjabi for sour face) and described my behaviour as *zidi* (meaning stubborn in Urdu). To her I had become some sort of miserable, pushy stubborn parent, a killjoy with a resting bitch face. I'd laugh to myself at this turnabout.

Aside from watching murder mystery reruns, I spent my time at her house flitting loosely about the kitchen, wondering what to make for our lunch and dinner. I always started with an onion – the basis of any good North Indian cuisine. I felt so connected to my memories of my time with my naniji, and her habitual cooking of the main meal in the morning to serve later in the day, and I felt like I was going through all the same processes and motions as my mum had as she cooked us our meals. I remembered wistfully all the steps of her methodical meal preparation and wondered how it had got to where we were today. I also thought about how much like an onion my mum's personality was. After her diagnosis, it was like we were peeling back a whole new layer and finding out so much more about her in the process. New parts of her life were coming into sharp focus as the outer layers were discarded; her earlier self, the inner core, was being revealed.

One thing I noticed was that when she talked about her childhood, it was as if she inhabited her body as a child. Her face changed and she somehow shone with a renewal of youth. It was like the memory was living in her and emanating from her, and she was watching the events play out in front of her eyes. She had travelled backwards through her history, but to her there was no sense of rewind. Instead she was seeing things as if they were happening for the first time.

My mother was born on the 19th January 1940 in Southport, England, but her parents swiftly returned to Bombay when she was a year or so old. One of the first things I learnt about Mum during 2017's long, summer evenings, sitting in her room when her soaps momentarily paused to allow a moment of silence, was that my naniji hadn't particularly liked her daughter, or at least that was what Mum had felt. Her mum, she would tell me, was desperate that her first child should be a boy, so when Asha came along there had been much disappointment. It was so strange for me to see my own feelings mirrored back to me in my mother, the woman who had made *me* feel like the disappointment my whole life, to learn that this was part of a generational trait inherited from *her* mother.

Our family was very North Indian culturally, and female infanticide in North India is still prevalent among some communities. Apparently daughters are takers not givers, and they continue to be seen in some parts as a burden on the family. Of course, it wasn't only mothers and daughters who had issues – all female relationships were defined by the lines drawn up by patriarchy. One of the stories Mum talked of was when her younger cousin came to live with them after Partition. Her father's brother's daughter arrived as an orphan, after both her parents had been killed in the horrific violence following the division of Punjab in 1947. For Aunty Thoshi it must have been a terrible time, but from Mum's retelling of the story, you could tell she had not liked her new companion because she had to share everything with another girl. Her position as the one girl in the household had been the only power she was afforded, albeit slight, and this was suddenly stripped away.

Mum often also talked about how her brothers were indulged by her mum, especially the youngest, who she was to fall out with so dramatically. He wasn't sent to boarding school like her other brothers, and by the time she was in her early teens Mum had the ability to really see the disparity in the way boys and girls were treated. Everybody put all their hopes and dreams into the boy-child, or at least that is what she felt her mother had done.

This revisionist history led me to see my grandmother in a different light. To me she had always been loving and caring, if set in her ways about how things should be done. Before she had dementia, Mum had only ever made vague comments about how she had felt about their relationship, but as her memories of that time began to return to the present, the heat of rejection stung afresh, finally enabling my mother to communicate her true feelings.

It led me to recall how, even after my grandmother had died, I'd been really surprised by the strength of her will. Even though her assets, the major financial things, had been split evenly between Mum and her brothers, when it had come to her personal possessions things were very different. Mum's job in the will had been to open the instructions for the bequests and to organize their delivery, but hardly any of my naniji's personal effects had been left to her at all.

I had always thought it strange, but I had never paid much attention to the idiosyncrasies within their relationship, or indeed why they remained even upon her mother's death. I hadn't realized that it had been based on a long-standing deep rift in their relationship. It never really occurred to me what sacrifice both women had made: Mum in coming to England again to forge a new life with her husband, and her mother letting her go to live thousands of miles away from her. The distance between them was both actual and metaphorical.

In a way, this led me to a greater understanding of my mum and of the difficulties our relationship had undergone over the years. It's hard to break a cycle; the way you experience love from a parent has an immense bearing on how you express love when a parent yourself. It's funny how even if you have felt the stab of injustice at rejection, that behaviour can still be passed on to the next generation. History repeats itself. For instance, the female grandchildren in my family believe that Akshay was spoilt by his grandmother, and up to a point I would agree with them. My mum did prefer boys, not that I think she was unfair to her female grandchildren. But it was just her natural preference, hammered deep into her, conditioned through culture and upbringing, until it was something immutable, the bedrock of her love.

Sometimes Mum described what she looked like and how she was dressed as the little girl she thought she was. She'd always be perfectly turned out, she would boast, in her red buckle school uniform, black polished shoes, white socks turned over just so and red ribbons in her hair. She'd then describe her long, gangly arms and legs and the almond shade of her summer skin. There would be tales of St Peter's School, Kandala, and she would sing a nursery rhyme learnt there: **'Pip pip pip pip tara rara rum, naney**

muney senek hum' – 'This is the way the soldiers walk early in the morning' – she'd trill as she skipped to school back in 1948. I would be told of St Anne's Convent School and her journeys there and back, catching the trains from Thakurli to Bombay all alone as a young child. Mum recited her three Hail Marys perfectly and regaled me with the same story of one of her teachers, Mother Sekoro, in her nun's attire, always ready with a pair of scissors to let down the hem of any skirt that was too short. Mum said she always worried about the inspection test, not because she was ever trying to show some leg, but because she was always growing and her mum, frugal as ever, wouldn't buy her a new skirt.

Mum recounted all the names of her childhood friends, telling me which ones were naughty, which ones were special to her. She remembered all the names of the nuns. She would talk about Aunty Vatsala, who was South Indian and had always got into trouble at school for her long and wavy untidy hair. Two of her favourite themes were how strict her parents were and their views around frugality and prudence – qualities which she had inherited and fostered in her own character. Budgeting, hating any kind of wastefulness and revelling in ingenious ways to either save money or reuse things were at the heart of lots of her stories, and I would listen to them for hours.

One minute I'd be sitting next to my eight-year-old mum, riding the railway to the convent chewing on Rowntree's fruit gums, then a TV theme tune would interject and her cogs would start to whir, taking us to another present that was happening at the same time as all the other pasts and the present she was living in. All at once. She'd remember a Beatles song if we were watching *Heartbeat* and begin to repeat the lines as if they were being transmitted through her, and then she would start describing Blackpool in such exquisite detail, because she had been to see The Beatles there with Dad. Then the focus would only be Blackpool, how it was baby Hema's favourite place, when she was a little child...that's why they were there, that's why they went. Imitating Hema, she'd ask, **'Are we going to Blackpool?'**, all wide-eyed and excited. She would then spend hours in the Blackpool in her mind, experiencing it once more afresh. The picnics on the beach. The fresh and windy sunshiny days. This might lead her on to thinking about Aunty Stella, who she'd stayed with, together with my Uncle Bill, when she first returned to England.

She loved telling any story where India came off better than England. She'd start by impressing you with how at home (India) she'd always loved biscuits and, even though her parents had been frugal, she'd been able to eat an unlimited number of those crumbly sweet treats. But when she came to stay with Uncle Bill and Aunty Stella, her biscuits were rationed. Mum keenly felt there was a difference between 'British' hospitality and 'Indian' hospitality. She never got over that her biscuits were measured out and that Aunty Stella would say, 'How many biscuits have you had? We are being greedy today, aren't we, Asha?' Mum would tell me how she had to bite her tongue, because of course you couldn't answer back to your hosts, it wasn't polite. Instead she'd recall how she would hide in her room and eat her hidden stash of Rich Tea.

Another day she would talk about the house she grew up in (I actually visited it once as part of a documentary called *Empire's Children*, although by then it was a shell of what it once was). In Mum's recollection it was a very beautiful bungalow in the colonial style, edged with a wonderful veranda. It had freestanding baths and plumbed-in toilets, a world away from the lean-to outside our first family home. She'd tell us her name at home was 'Baby'. As her parents were well-to-do, they had house help and an ayah, so it was all, **'Baby, what do you want to drink?**

Baby, here are your clothes today.' She didn't grow up doing any housework, she'd whisper that her family were posh. Then suddenly we would skip forward to the pubs my grandad used to like around Bolton, the Beehive being the place where he had his first alcoholic drink. Then she'd move on to how the only reason her parents could drink tea in England when she was born was because they received milk rations as she was a baby.

Keeping track of where Mum was – or more accurately which version of Mum she was at any point – could be exhausting. It felt like her memory was a singular chain in which the links had been broken, put into a bag and shaken up, then randomly reassembled in an order that made no sense to anyone.

Most of the time Mum didn't see me as a woman standing before her – instead she saw me as my teenage self, the child who needed discipline, who had been the third disappointment in a row and was always a mess. **'You mean you went to the chemist with that hair, Shobna?'** she'd say aghast, questioning how I could possibly have left the house looking like that. Our present just wasn't her focus; she stopped living in our shared moment.

She had always been full of advice and reprimand, but now she often wasn't plugged in to things going on around her. The strange thing is that the past was available to her with such immediacy and clarity that there was no question of her not feeling as though she was experiencing it all, then and there, before you.

We think about dementia as being out of step with the present, and it is, but only if we're talking about our 'shared' perception of the present. Mum didn't know she was combing back through her history – she was living whatever was playing through her head as though time held no power. She was so startlingly close to all of her memories that it was as though they were all playing at once like a complex piece of jazz, and I would have to focus on the individual story like I would on one instrument. It's all a question of perspective. She became an all-seer who saw past the limitations of our dimensions. She could see so far beyond our limits. Of course, dark patches had grown too within her memory, which meant they were for ever erased from her mind. It was as though someone had gone into her filing cabinet and locked away certain periods, people, present happenings and she would never again find the keys. But perhaps who you are isn't really about what you forget, but what you remember. As Mum became unfixed from essential details of her life, she was free to go into herself even further, alone and unencumbered.

CHAPTER SEVEN

What are you waiting for?

In every relationship I've had I've struggled to form boundaries and maintain them. I can only presume it originated in my early need for validation. I was prepared to forgo my needs and wants, to erase myself, in order to fit in. I learnt early on to become entirely mutable, adapting every facet of myself to the person I was with; progressing from my mother and father to my siblings and then to my peers. Whoever I was with, I never carved out space that didn't include them in order to try to find balance in my own life. I have always allowed the needs of others to subsume and consume mine.

As the caring months headed towards years, I did as I have always done, and I shifted my everything to fit around and centre on my mother. Everything became about Asha Gulati to the detriment of pretty much any other thing in my life. In fact, I never put any thought into when I would focus on my own life or pick its needs back up.

It was just indefinite. An indefinite pause.

I would rush through my life admin, ballsing it all up in the process, because I was trying to squeeze it into another's timetable. I was late to respond to emails, including work opportunities. Messages and calls from my agent and friends went unanswered. I never paid my bills on time, so I was constantly being charged overdue fees. I stopped opening my post because that could wait, so whenever I did make it back to my house on a Wednesday evening, there would be these mountains of envelopes that had piled up. My life too seemed to pile up on the doormat of my mind, never making its way beyond it, remaining a peripheral feature, or at worst a source of administrative irritation that I would put off until the very last moment.

The stress of last-minute living became overwhelming. I had responsibilities to charities and organizations, and I let these obligations slip away bit by bit too. I couldn't compartmentalize looking after my mother – and I never felt able to bring my own life into her home and try and organize it from there.

Without realizing it, I chose to sacrifice the outside world. It was how I coped. Blocking out the world around us and focusing on Mum meant I blinkered myself from the everyday stresses and strains and that helped me to keep the sense of overwhelm at bay. It was as if I too had started using a permanent marker to scribble out and censor sections of my memory which I couldn't hold on to any more. Anything I couldn't deal with was just cut off.

I'd even draw a blank with picking up the phone – I had nothing to say to anyone. 'Yes, I'm still here with Mum, nothing has changed.' Literally nothing in months. Literally nothing in years. I stopped knowing how to talk to my friends. How to talk to myself and care for myself. Everything except Mum was lost.

For any carer in a similar situation, finding room for a partner or keeping up friendships is nigh on impossible. When I wasn't working, I was sitting watching telly with Mum. I couldn't properly date or go on long holidays to rest from work, or meet my friends regularly. I wasn't building a life any more.

During the early days of caring for Mum I had been involved with a man, who I had thought might be the partner I could share the rest of my life with. His mum had been ill too – she sadly passed away while we were together. But it didn't work out. It had ended acrimoniously and with no closure, and I was angry and sad. I had not been present enough to notice the red flags in the relationship and, as a parting shot, he had cruelly said, 'Go and look after your mum.' As if she had been the reason he had decided to disappear. The next thing I knew he had replaced me with a brand new relationship.

I couldn't absorb anything, I had no room or time to process my feelings, but I couldn't stop crying. Mum kept looking at me, but she didn't say anything, then suddenly she asked, **'What is wrong, Shobna?'** I remember saying that it was a sad programme on the telly, but she kept prodding me again and again, **'No, no, no, no, no. There's something wrong. What is it? You're crying.'** In that instant I was both comforted by the fact that she still 'knew' something was wrong and anguished that I wouldn't be really able to explain it to her fully. That she didn't have the cognitive process she once had to make things better. Instead, I managed to change the subject and then inevitably she forgot.

I desperately wished that she could help me, like she had at other times in our life together, but I knew that she couldn't. I found that so sad and so hard. While I have always had terrible romantic relationships, she was constantly there to give me advice, usually in the car. I had invariably made a point of introducing her to each of them in order to get her approval, and her judgement had been spot on with every single one of the suitors she had met. She was also full of her usual tough love. She wouldn't wax lyrical, or spend hours listening to me on the phone, her assessments would always be short, succinct and smart.

I remember her asking me once why I was crying over yet another break up: **'Why are you so upset, Shobna?'** she said. **'That man lives in a room in a house. Darling, you're a homeowner.'**

As soon as I hit my forties, in her mind I was on the shelf for any happily-ever-afters. Not that she didn't want to meet my boyfriends and mete out her judgement, but she now felt that I'd had my time and I should find happiness in staying single, just as she had. But we were different in that way, I still held out hope that I would meet someone to share my life with. And now, as I sat next to my mother, crying over that man in whom I had invested what little spare time I had in between caring for her, I was desperate for those words of advice. But I knew at this stage I couldn't explain to her what had happened. From this point onwards, anything I experienced emotionally I would go through all by myself. In the grand scheme of caring and being with Mum it didn't really matter, and the hurt eventually went, but the loneliness continued to creep into me as the memories inched out of Mum.

I began to exist only in a tiny bubble oscillating between Mum's house and ASDA, Tesco, M&S for a 'fancy' treat, and the Worldwide Cash and Carry.

On the road to work,

at work,

on the road back to Mum.

What I needed was for it all to stop, to spend a week in my own house straightening things out and time to gain some perspective. But I never managed to find that space for myself and I just sank deeper and deeper into caring for her without acknowledging myself.

I stopped brushing my hair and brushing my teeth. Mum would laugh at me and say, **'Shobna, what is this hair, you haven't brushed it!'** and I'd think, Well, I've brushed yours, Mum, and put your lipstick on and arranged for you to have your nails done at home by my friend Becky. I didn't get to consider myself. The truth is that I began to completely lose myself in being a carer. I didn't care about myself, I had no time or even desire to do that. I lost as much of my day-to-day life as Mum's memory erased of hers.

It became hard to define the passing of time as I cared for her. We were existing in stasis, as the days and months segued into each other. The fact that we were indoors so much, in her living room, where she also slept, compounded the feeling of incarceration – it was the sense that we had stopped our lives as the carnival of life raged outside. In my attempts to try and get a handle on time, I started to keep notes of the daily minutiae; records of appointments or tracking the rare outings. I wrote down the stories that she began to share too.

Before Mum woke up, I noted in my phone the different things that were on my mind. I'd silently go downstairs, slip into the small front room where she slept and turn off her television. Then I'd go back upstairs to my childhood bedroom, and sit in bed and type all the things she had revealed to me about her life, the things that she had remembered or wanted to tell me, everything that had come up the day before. I wrote every detail I could recall in a stream of consciousness, uninterrupted.

I was trying to make sense of things; I'd reorganize our experiences. I'd write poems and then try to bend them into a linear path, as otherwise it would be a gallimaufry of meals, medical appointments, social or religious events. The repetitive routine was unhinged from any other markers of passing time. There were no tent poles to fasten the chronology of her thoughts to, so I tried to restore them into an order each and every morning.

I would WhatsApp the 'Team Mum Care' group, made up of my siblings and my son, to update them on how she slept, what she ate, what mood she had been in – 'prickly' or in 'good' humour – whether she was physically well or if there any changes in her breathing or swelling in her feet, ankles, fingers or legs. I enjoyed regaling the group with lengthy descriptions of the food I had cooked, which would read like something from a Michelin starred restaurant menu.

Most weeks would pass without peaks or troughs – life flatlined. Mum sitting on her bed, propped up by an array of cushions, me on the big black leather reclining armchair, watching the same murder mystery rerun on the telly for the 14th time...Like Mum's messages to St Anthony desperate to keep hold of her possessions, my notes and thoughts on my phone helped me keep hold of time. And just as she had secretly been ordering and recording all the press clippings of my life, I began to do the same for her.

Outside of my diary, the only clearly traceable aspect of her decline could be found by tracking the rooms we were sleeping in. When I first started staying over, in 2015, I slept in a single bed in the room that had been Akshay's during the years Mum had cared for him. It was a pain and a half, because that childhood bed did my back right in. I mean, it felt like it was centuries old by this point, but I just made do. I never raised it as I knew my mother would have had something to say about me buying a new bed when there was one still standing. Then, as I became a regular overnight visitor, in an admission that my role as Mum's carer was becoming more permanent, I moved into my own childhood bedroom, which had been redecorated and refurnished by Sushma when she was living and working in Oldham before her marriage. Despite replacing my mattress at my own home, for about five years I rarely slept in my own bed.

Sometime earlier, in 2013, so before her bowel cancer diagnosis, Mum had said she wanted her bed moved downstairs. It wasn't such a surprise as climbing the staircase had become a struggle and she'd huff and puff and be unsteady on her feet as her mobility had taken a hit. But leaving behind her marital bedroom and the double bed felt as though she was parting with the person she had been for most of her life, both before my father died when they were a couple and then after he died as his widowed wife. Her marriage had been the cornerstone of *her* identity and this move downstairs, even if the distance was no more than six feet below, ushered in a schism that had now become vast. As she made that transition, it somehow seemed to cut a tie with her past, and her recollections of her old adult self slowly started to be blotted out, superseded by tableaux of her youth.

We had set her up with huge cushions for her back, in front of her beloved TV, as she didn't like sitting on chairs, and we put her bed next to the radiator to keep her cosy. Soon she was rarely going upstairs, except to shower. On occasion she'd go up to find a bag of papers or else come back down and say she couldn't remember what had inspired her to scale the treads in the first place. In the not so distant past she used to love doing the laundry and the ironing – the utility room was upstairs, and the ironing board and iron positioned comfortably in front of another widescreen television in her bedroom. This had always been her routine, to do the ironing while watching her TV and then meticulously fold up all the pressed linen, putting everything away, neatly. But by this point she had completely stopped. Unwashed laundry had piled up. The iron and board stayed up against the wall like a museum exhibit. And, as she wasn't one to go for a walk, the four walls of her downstairs bedroom quickly became the parameters of her world.

We had all been brought up to believe that we had a cultural responsibility and duty to our family until the very end, no ifs nor buts. The fact that there are so many elderly people in homes in Britain is something that most families in our community judge harshly, and it's the reason you are less likely to find many of us in residential or care homes. A home just wasn't a consideration for us. It's about looking after each other within the parameters of the extended family. As the younger generation, we were honour-bound to care for our elders.

Back in my parents' day, when some women didn't work outside the home, there would be a small army of women at home or nearby available to care for older relatives. Shared among daughters, daughters-in-law, countless granddaughters and the regular home help some middle-class families employed, this practice of dividing the labour for caring can work. But in the here and now, working women from my community are expected to uphold the same levels of caring in situations that have become much more complicated.

Strictly speaking, within our cultural patriarchy, care of elderly parents should lie with the eldest son and his wife – just one of the reasons why sons are given so much value. As my dad was the chosen child, it was expected that my mum, all those years ago in Mumbai, would look after her in-laws in their dotage. However, it was left to my uncle and aunt – the younger brother and his wife – due to the geographical distance and the fact that my mum had a family to raise here. This could have been seen as an abdication of duty, no matter what the circumstances. These indoctrinated attitudes are still in place and the responsibility still unfairly rests solely on the women – daughters and daughters-in-law who make up a family – even though so many of us work and earn good salaries. Even if they live thousands of miles away, the responsibility is theirs. No matter how society has changed, the responsibility is theirs.

Among my close Indian, Bangladeshi, Pakistani and Sri Lankan friends, who were mostly born here, nearly all of us had become carers. Privately, to one another, we could express our feelings that it was all too much, and discuss the guilt that came with that. Publicly, we got on with the job – we were all complicit, as we all understood what was expected of us and accepted it. I suppose it's similar to the way in which women who work full-time are also expected to somehow 'have it all' and look after their children as well. You could feel deeply guilty if you didn't live up to these expectations. At some point you have to choose.

I knew all along I was the one within my family with a debt to repay, and it was presumed that whenever I wasn't working I would be with Mum. In those early days, the only time off I had, aside from when I was working, was when Raj covered Wednesday nights and Thursday mornings. That gave me a few hours' break, and it was the only time I'd get home to my own bed. I had brought my own duvet and pillow over to Mum's, so on Wednesday I'd stuff them back into a bin liner and take them home. I lived for those one-off nights in my own bed. Those years, I hardly sat down, I was either at Mum's beck and call, or racing up and down the motorway trying to fit work in, or halfway across the country or rushing back to be there for her.

One of the biggest issues of my career, and something that lots of freelancers will recognize, is the unpredictability of work. Sometimes you hit a great run and you're flush, other times work can be really sparse. Combining that with being a carer was basically impossible. Caring is a full-time job, you can't just dip in and out of it, so trying to earn any consistent money was a struggle. I'd find myself trying to schedule several auditions at once, so I could come down to London for a day and then make it back for Mum. Trying to get anything done at her house was really hard – forget learning lines or even trying to sort out the practicalities of a 'self tape' (an audition on video). All day long I'd be up and down, every time she called for me. You couldn't just leave her, but there wouldn't be a break. From the moment Mum woke up to when she went to sleep you never knew what would happen next.

There was no regular routine, but a typical day could look like this: Mum woke late and then went to the bathroom. While she was in there, I sorted her room out – made her bed, prepped her breakfast and maybe even did a quick hoover up and thorough wipe down of the surfaces. I replaced undrunk water with a fresh cup. Essentially, Mum still had an absolute conviction in not only her ability but also her domestic pride. I didn't want to run the risk of a row over how I was cleaning, but I also wanted her to think she'd done it all herself. Asha was still a formidable force and kept her house tidy and cooked everyone's meals, thank you very much.

Mum would appear from the bathroom, sometimes with a jolly step (if she'd slept long enough). **'I've had my beauty sleep,'** she'd joke, then to cheer her along, with a smile I'd say, 'Tea?' At that magic word, her face lit up and she'd say, **'Please, I've brushed my teeth,'** and flash me a grin to show just how clean and bright her smile was. 'Mum, it's all cosy, sit here, I'll bring your tea,' I'd say, and accompany her back to her bed, where I'd put a warm wheat bag on her cushions, to make sure she wouldn't sit herself by the radiator. **'Ooo that's nice,'** she'd say.

I couldn't then say, 'I'm learning lines, I've got stuff to do' to someone who has dementia. You can't say, 'Can you hurry along so I can get on with it?' How would that make sense when they don't inhabit the same world any more? To be fair, it's hard enough explaining the nature of an actor's life to anyone outside of the industry, let alone someone struggling to remember their place in the world.

There was a lot I had to be attentive to, to ensure everything was done correctly. But there was also a lot of waiting. One of the things I waited around for were her moments of lucidity. You never knew when a story would materialize and present itself within your conversation. If I could get a conversation going about her life, and sit prompting her with questions, she could begin to tell tales I'd never heard before, and that was incredibly precious. I'd really love all the unusual names of her St Anne's schoolfriends, Indian Catholic girls' names, like Blossom Sanchez and Jocelyn Mascarenhas. I'd note them down as Mum remembered their personalities. Her early life was filled with rainbow colours and she was totally enchanted with her memories, as was I; they entertained and delighted us day to day.

We carried on watching *a lot* of TV together. She still loved her soaps, the news and her mystery dramas. She got really into

Hercule Poirot, and loved David Suchet's surprise and exasperation with English ways. She would laugh out loud and regale me with some story about the strangeness of Anglo-Saxon culture and its unfathomable idiosyncrasies. **'That's the English,'** she would say, **'how can "spotted dick" ever be delicious?'** and we would laugh, Mum knowing she had said something controversial and naughty – you could see it in the mischief in her eyes.

Sometimes, something would come on and Mum would have an opinion on it, and although we had stopped being able to have everyday chats about normal life, we were able to talk about anything as long as it was exactly wherever her mind was at that moment. I began to get glimpses of my mum which I'd never seen before. Sometimes when I put her to bed, she smiled in a way that I couldn't recognize, as though she was a pre-schooler being tucked up, and those brief windows into her previous selves made every minute of caring for her worth it.

When we settled down to watch *Coronation Street*, she would quizzically ask me about my character Sunita when she spotted a picture of me in the back of shot. **'Are you dead?'** she'd ask. And I'd say, 'Yes, Mum, on the programme I am. Do you remember? You cried when my character died?' Seeing a framed photograph of a loved one indicated culturally to her that someone had died. Her own home was filled with mounted pictures of numerous late relatives. I'd try to make light of the situation, and say, 'It doesn't matter that I'm dead, Mum, your legacy lives on', and I'd remind her that Sunita named her daughter, Asha, after her. That pleased her no end. She would always be part of the history of her beloved *Coronation Street*.

But it was confusing, and sometimes the only release was to empty my mind of the random thoughts, good or bad, whatever had happened in the day. I simply wrote my immediate thoughts down. It was a form of release.

She was sleeping
time was keeping
weighing
preying on her mind

What would she find
in her dreams
could she know what they mean?

Passing thoughts
we fought
this morning
I heard her
a warning
that things were not right for her
I had to fight for her
She had every ounce of dignity
without clear lucidity
I could only practically help
the ninja stealth of my negotiations
Yesterday she asked me what was prorogation
Whimsical laugh/she's not daft
She's still there/it's not fair
She's asleep now
I'm just working out how
I can help her when she wakes
It's all give and not take
That's the passage of time
In my basic rhymes

In the early days we could leave Mum alone for a few hours with the cameras we'd installed, and keep an eye on her. As long as I'd left food and written instructions, and Raj could pop in to check on her now and then, she would be OK. She was still able to navigate her room, the kitchen and her bathroom. She never did anything risky or went wandering off – there is no such thing as identikit dementia, each individual has an entirely unique experience and Mum had hers. That means also there's no pamphlet or internet research that can prepare you for how a person deteriorates, the pace of their memory's evaporation or what will be left behind. So, while I didn't worry about Mum suddenly absconding or burning the house down, and the car had been disconnected so there was no more fear around that, I was very concerned whenever I had any long stints working, that Mum would deteriorate quickly in my absence.

Now that I knew what was really going on, I felt guilty, desperately guilty, about having been away for work in those years before her diagnosis was clear. If I'd been there more would I have noticed more? Perhaps I'd have paid more attention to my concerns? I obviously suspected that there was something more serious than she was letting on, but I didn't speak up enough and I still think about that a lot. Gradually, gradually, gradually everything became more pronounced, more symptomatic. The condition built and built but of course we didn't really know it was building, because we hadn't determined, right at the onset, that it even existed.

If I had to travel for work at that time, Sushma came up from Hertford to look after her. I often found solace in my professional life – it became my relief and sanctuary, in some ways allowing me to escape the prism of care, emancipating me from my daily duties. But it was also hugely stressful, because I was going up and

down the country constantly trying to keep my career professional
while also trying desperately to cover the care. If I was working in
the theatre, sometimes I'd take the night bus from central London
on a Saturday at midnight. It went via Luton Airport all around
the houses until it reached Chorlton Street, Manchester at 5.30am.
I would go straight to Mum's by taxi, where I'd try and get a couple
of hours of sleep and then have the full day on Sunday looking
after her. At some point during the day, I'd do the food shop and
all the cooking for the week ahead, putting it all into labelled
containers in the fridge. Then I packed up and went straight back
down to London for a week of work, starting with an evening show
on the Monday, without ever crossing my doorstep.

Even though we all played our parts in the care of our mum, the
differences in our methods and ways of caring for her sometimes
caused conflict between my siblings and me. Coupled with pre-
existing tensions, we found it hard to not let all this build up and
spill over. We were scared, we were lost without her, we loved
her and we were handling it in increasingly different ways. The
pressure that caring for a parent with dementia can put on your
relationships with your family is immense. It's one of the reasons
that Raj, Hema and I are now estranged.

   This strain is one of the things that no one talks about – it isn't
addressed by our overstretched but compassionate healthcare
workers or bullet-pointed in leaflets. Family tensions aren't
discussed in the public domain. But a vast amount of negotiation
has to go on when a family begins to care for one of its members,
and you have to dig deep to become a happy family and a united
team, especially when you aren't to start with.

   It takes a toll on everyone. All of your lives, your relationships
and past grievances are part of this negotiation of care. They

can't be sidestepped or overlooked, instead they are intrinsic counters in how you weigh up who will step forward and provide the primary care. It's not just the endless WhatsApps and the drawing up of the calendar. The who-will-do-what, the splitting of responsibilities and areas of duty. It's also about your differing natures and your individual ways of being a carer and the conflict that can engender. The 'Oh I do that this way', and the sense of judgement you can feel about your choices, especially the ones you make under pressure. You have to be incredibly kind to each other and empathize at every corner, or else blame and recrimination can seep in. The fallout that caring can have on your family dynamic just can't be underestimated. Somehow, I did not know how to ask for a break or a holiday and I felt that I had to explain why my work mattered, or why I might need a breather. Rightly or wrongly, I felt judged and I felt incredible guilt over any rest period.

In 2017, I was anxious after a pretty patchy year work-wise, so I signed up to do a Christmas theatre show. The job was fringy, which meant that it had a great director and was very well respected, but also that the wages were fringy too. I think it paid £300 a week before commission. My agent had said that it wouldn't harm me to go into it for a bit of reinvention. People would see me in a different light and it would remind them I could do proper theatre, not just the commercial stuff that paid a commercial salary. It was only for six weeks.

When it was settled that I was going, I felt that I had to calculate exactly how much time I was going to be away. I would still be coming back for Sundays and some Mondays, which we had off, and to look after Mum's shopping and cooking where required. But that wasn't the point. I felt that some members of the family, especially my brother, thought it was my job to be with

Mum no matter what the sacrifice to my career. I had to know how many hours out of my 'real' job I was taking and how those hours would impact him and the rest of the family.

Raj played his own role in caring, as he was medically skilled. Helping to liaise with doctors and nurses over the upkeep of Mum's health, he was always the person Mum would eventually listen to about medication and about her health. In many ways he took on the role that my dad had, as doctor. Mum knew the story of that relationship and was often more comfortable with taking advice from my brother. Raj was great at the appointments he attended with Mum, and organizing things for her and keeping up with all the medical jargon which sometimes went over my head. He would also, on occasion, tackle some of her personal admin. But his temperament just wasn't suited to the long carer's hours. He lacked the sustained patience of the day-in and day-out stamina it took, and he had the pressure of his own family too.

Of course, we all lost our rag from time to time because it could be incredibly intense, and Mum could often be infuriating – she liked to do things in her own way in her own time and refused to admit at any point she was incapable of doing certain things. I did everything in my power to avoid confrontation, because I didn't want to upset her, and I also didn't want to put that extra stress on myself. But no one is superhuman, and when your patience is tried time and time again, right to its very edge, it's impossible to keep perfectly calm every single day. I would snap, and fight back – just with words, I hasten to add. Afterwards I'd feel desperately guilty about what I had said and tussle with my conscience about having told her 'you do it then', as it was invariably a struggle between what she thought she could do and what sadly she really couldn't.

I'd escape to my bedroom but, instead of trying to relax, I'd be thinking, Why did I do that? I couldn't shake it off, I'd blame myself and wonder when the best time would be to go back down, as if I had acted like the naughty teenage Shobna and I had been answering back. We are all caught in the net of who our family thought we once were and the people we are today. Of course, by the time I made it back down the stairs she'd have forgotten it all – there would be no trace of the tension I had escaped from, as though she had cleaned it all away while I had my back turned, hoovered it all up and tidied it all back to order.

Like most actors, I've had to contend with others' ideas that my job is 'a bit of fun', rather than a real job, and doesn't really count as a career. That's across the board. It's certainly my family's response. If I'd been a schoolteacher or a lawyer or an accountant, it may have made the balancing act easier. I got the sense that sometimes siblings felt I was off on a holiday when I was down in London working. It's as if the job I do isn't real, isn't hard, isn't a challenge. But, you know, just because I enjoy my job , doesn't mean that it's not work. Just because my work appears glamorous, it doesn't mean it isn't backbreaking too. I love what I do, but it's certainly not all roses.

Think about what you see at the theatre – as a member of the audience you have these gorgeous, deep red plush velvet chairs. You go to the bar and drink the drinks and eat the food and you watch the amazing spectacle, and your whole evening feels like a luxury. But backstage it's grim. Sometimes theatres don't have working toilets or showers, there will be no sinks, no soap, and you'll find all sorts of rubbish and rodents backstage. Sometimes we'll all be squashed into one dressing room, cheek by jowl. The hours are long and arduous. And yes, of course you have a laugh from time to time because, my God, you need it. But enjoying your work doesn't mean that it is somehow less valuable, or less exhausting or stressful.

Acting isn't seen as a respectable profession by my community. And, of course, everyone presumed I wasn't respectable either. Shobna Gulati was never respectable from start to finish because, in the eyes of certain people, including those in my family, I had been guilty of 'demanding that my mum looked after my son and me'. Judgement would resurface whenever I had to work; there was no recognition that I had my mortgage and bills to pay like everybody else, and I had to look after my son.

I had long stints without being cast, which meant there were times when I was broke and cash was really tight. Some of the feedback was crushing. Where do I start? Some directors said I didn't look 'Asian enough', some that I looked 'too Asian'. (Of course, these criticisms were always from white casting directors and white producers.) With others I wasn't taken seriously because I hadn't had formal drama school training, without any thought given to how difficult it is to access that kind of education as a Black or Brown person. We all know the game is rigged and even as a well-known and successful British actress of Indian heritage, finding consistent work has been a huge challenge. My late former agent once said that because I mostly played 'middle-aged victims' I would invariably end up on a casting director's list 'as the last "n-word" in the woodpile'. It's horrific, and what's most shocking is that this casually delivered racism is symptomatic of just another day living as a woman of colour in this country. That's serious shit.

Then there is the generalized belief, which I have encountered time and time again that being an actor on *Coronation Street* 'makes you for life'. This is a myth. The money was regular and the years of working on *Coronation Street* took the financial pressure off. It enabled me to buy my home and to pay to send

Akshay to grammar school and then to a performing arts school, after he gained a part-scholarship. But when my character was killed off, it was back to the old ways of sporadic work, and there wasn't some huge pot of savings to tide me through the tough times. My new agents and I were locked in a constant fight with casting directors who said I would 'only ever be Sunita'. This idea that I couldn't play other roles was the prejudice and bias I faced regularly, but whenever I mentioned this to some of my white colleagues I'd be told I was being 'chippy'.

As it felt I was encountering one brick wall after another, I decided to focus on short commercial jobs, where the audience would love to watch 'someone famous', to make sure I was earning the maximum amount of money in the shortest amount of time. So whenever I was away from Mum, it would be worth it. This of course had an impact on the future roles I was offered, and the ones I chose. Most well-regarded theatre work isn't particularly well paid. 'What are you doing it for then?' was an unsaid but implied question from many. But sometimes I needed to take those jobs to show the wider acting world what I was capable of, in order to open up other opportunities. So much to do all the time, this pressure to prove prove prove yourself to everyone. It was and is very hard to cope with the blood, sweat, tears and fight required to build an acting career, particularly when it's given such little respect. What was clear was that the conflict between my career and caring was my problem to solve.

As I was looking after Mum more and more, the window between my professional life and my life as a carer began to close. I had to find a way of keeping it ajar, even if only slightly, to keep my life aerated and offer me some doses of reality even if at erratic intervals. Finally, in early 2018, aged 51, I got my first role in the West End, London's prestigious home of theatre and musical theatre, playing Ray in *Everybody's Talking About Jamie*. Mum said, **'It's what you have always wanted and dreamt of since you first started dancing.'** She was right, it was very important to me.

In the end, the only thing I could think to do was turn to another woman in my home community for help with Mum's care. Jayshri was an old friend – our kids had gone to school together locally and, because my mum had been Akshay's guardian, she knew her well too. With Gujarati heritage, Jayshri had a wonderful sensibility of how Mum might be about certain things. She'd also worked in social care for years and had cared for her own mum until she sadly lost her to vascular dementia. Since her mother had recently passed away, she was doing odd bits here and there in order to get back into work, and I asked if she'd like to join our 'Team Mum Care' on a paid basis. Fortunately, she said yes. She was fantastic, and would make Mum delicious meals free of charge. She was the tonic that everyone needed.

It worked out well – my mum absolutely loved her. Before I left for London to start the job, Jayshri, Mum and I would regularly meet for a cup of tea and a chat. Before long Jayshri was no longer just my friend, but my mum's too. I can still picture Mum sitting there cosied up on the cushions, saying, **'Put the kettle on, let's share the tasty treats my friend Jayshri has brought.'**

When I returned home to Mum after working, my social life was nonexistent. At Mum's, aside from struggling to speak to friends on the phone, I saw no one. I didn't go to the cinema or restaurants. I didn't hear music or drink a glass or two in a pub. I didn't even make it to Manchester for years. On one rare occasion when I met a friend in town for the Manchester Festival, I didn't recognize the city at all! I couldn't read the skyline or remember the streets; I didn't know where to go for food or a coffee. I had become a tourist in my own city. I also felt lost and guilty just being there. My isolation, both social and geographic, had a massive impact on my mental health. The doors were shut even tighter on our little front room. Anything that wasn't Mum just didn't have a chance.

Watching the way my sister Sushma managed her time with Mum highlighted how the situation could have been different for me. Sushma, the middle sister, had always been the diplomat of the family, the arbiter whenever the peace was broken. She is a very balanced woman. Even though her work and family life were really impacted by Mum's illnesses, as she had to travel up from her family home in Hertford, sometimes with her husband, Søren, who became part of Team Mum, she always found a way to try and keep things on an even keel. She would bring things to do with her, things from her own life and only for herself, but often these remained in the boot of her car for the whole visit. She admitted to me that sometimes even she was unable to find those slivers of personal time, as things with Mum could always change. But every day, without fail, she would take a walk and get outside, which definitely helped break the spell when the tension within the four walls ratcheted up. She'd channel her energies into doing a 'big clean' to keep order and uphold Mum's values of being houseproud while also being available for her, and in that way she dealt with the pressure and yet kept herself occupied with her own aims and goals, even if they were focused within Mum's home.

The sacred space of our mother's kitchen would lead to all sorts of confrontation and drama, but as time passed, Mum's ways and her worries around her kitchen started to dissolve. The instructions on how to make tea which had been drilled into us since childhood stopped being barked from a distance.

**She stopped checking on your technique before she
countenanced her first sip.
She stopped checking if you had used the teapot.
She stopped asking if you had put in two bags, not three.
She didn't care if the water was filled up to the top hole.
She didn't ask where you'd put the used tea bag.
She didn't force you to bring the pot over to her to check.**

Even though she forgot a lot of her peculiarities, she always
remembered that she couldn't eat aubergines and when I'd
cook her a vegetable sabji, she would say, **'I don't eat Baingan
(aubergine). You didn't put any in, did you?'** (Then she would
always make a wry joke that my sister-in-law was really an 'outlaw'
as Raj's wife eats aubergines despite the Gulati rule. Though now, I
hasten to add, we're not bothered. We are not the aubergine police!)

Then came the point when Mum stopped wanting to get
physically involved with the food and drink preparation, which
was shocking to us all. We had all been micromanaged within an
inch of a vegetable chop and suddenly it passed her by as though
she had never really minded at all. The way she wanted you to
boil the potatoes before you peeled them by hand, painstakingly
scratching off the skin bit by bit, so you didn't waste any of the
potato flesh, the specific angle you had to cut an onion or even
to peel it to ensure you didn't lose any of it – all of these irritating
eccentricities began to disappear from her, and her requests
and the standards she had always held us all to began to slip.
Gradually, I started cooking for Mum in her own house and
gradually she stopped checking on every little thing I was doing.
The one thing that didn't disappear was her matriarchal focus
on her dominion, which led to her believing that she had cooked
and prepared every meal we had made and was also running

the house by herself. It was an incredibly bizarre development and became difficult to manage – as even though she was hardly getting up from her cushions, she believed that she had put the washing machine on and folded and ironed all the clothes, as well as having cooked the meals we were eating. She thought she had cleaned the house and organized her daily life around her. Sometimes she thought she'd made the tea. But she hadn't – we'd done it all.

We in turn kept up this charade as we didn't know how else to handle her absolute conviction not only in her ability but also her domestic pride. This semblance of still being in control absolutely made her feel more secure and it also meant that the giant gaps in her care never took place. But I worried that I was disabusing her of the truth. I never corrected her and told her, 'Mum, no, you didn't make the tea; no, you didn't make the dinner. I did.' How do you say that to someone who stridently is holding onto their independence, at least trying to preserve it in their mind, as a way of offsetting the devastating effects her degeneration was having on her character, her activity, her pride?

I began to disguise the manual work I was undertaking so as not to dislodge her belief in her capabilities. When Mum would go to the toilet – I would begin to hoover and then once that was done, I would end up being able to change the bed, put a wash on and then do another quick once-over with the hoover before she came out. I didn't want to run the risk of a row over how I was cleaning, but I also wanted her to think she'd done it all herself.

The Asha standards of how to run a house slowly became a thing of the past. Appearances were no longer kept up and it was as though a gushing tap was turned off. Droplets continued to drip out regularly to begin with, but slowly the normal flow of rituals and benchmarks we had to keep to were released from her mind.

She dried up. The day Mum stopped ironing, or walked into the kitchen and made a cup of mug tea were the moments I realized we would never get her tap running again. It was just the kind of defining characteristic and peculiarity that made her *her*. All these rules, all these Gulati yardsticks that my siblings and I laughed at and rolled our eyes over, my God I missed them all so deeply when they were gone.

Caring is time-consuming and often bleeds into all-consuming. There is a lot of drudgery in its repetitive nature. You don't have the expectation that it will be just for a few days or weeks, you know that this will continue for years of your life. And there is nothing tangible created in this space. It's not like early motherhood, where things are constantly moving forward, where even in the daily drudgery there is always progress. To fill the space, I began to channel a lot of my energies into cooking for my mum – this felt less about staving off entropy for another day and more about nurturing and creation. I cooked to perk Mum up and bring some joy into her day.

As I was chopping the onion that I always started with, I'd decide which powdered spices and which whole spices I would use, and that would determine the dish. I'd add whichever vegetables were left in the fridge. I'd make biryani from leftover curries and throw in the frozen veg from steam bags in the freezer to make the flavourful rice dish more vibrant. But there were also fish finger sandwiches, where I'd melt butter into peas and mash them into the bread to make a bed for the crispy fish – Mum always loved 'green bread', and would laugh whenever I made it for her because it looked so uninviting. She found that funny. Like everything in our life, it was a mix of north of England and our North Indian flavours.

Mum's favourite meals consisted of anything to do with potatoes, or 'aloos', the affectionate English plural of the Hindi word for spud. She loved aloos mashed, boiled, baked, in an Indian mixed-veg stir-fry, or subji, or cooked in a dry 'Bombay' style, with cumin seeds and turmeric. Mum had a massive thing for chips and she'd always be sending Akshay up to the chippy for a bag or two, though she'd be happy as a clam with homemade too. Other favourites included a South Indian dish combining a spicy, dry mix of masala potatoes and cooked onions stuffed into dosas (Sushma often brought a handy readymade dosa pancake mix to make for Mum). Mum loved potato chaat (mashed potatoes seasoned with lemon, pepper, black salt, amchur/mango powder, chilli powder and garam masala in a spicy finger-licking chaat mix) mixed with a fried namkeen teatime snack. Other fail-safes were aloo tomato 'gravy', aloo matter (potato and peas), aloo saag (potato and spinach), potatoes stuffed into peppers (one of her Nirmala Niketan specials).

'Casey's potatoes', a creamy cheesy potato bake with chopped coloured peppers and nutmeg, was a dish she used to whip together for 'bring a dish' charity 'international food evenings'. Like me, she loved to subvert the stereotype and instead of an Indian dish she'd bring this American-style fare for the charity ladies, and why not? The absolute winner though was always aloo gobi (potato and cauliflower) which she would affectionately call gobi Shobi, laughing every time at her own joke.

I deliberately prepared certain meals to provoke lost memories and stories. Taste would reconnect her to her history. For instance, the taste of the rendered crispy fat on lamb cutlets would transport her to India, and she would giggle that the sheep must have been skinny as there was not much of this tasty treat. I soon learnt that cooking smells would make her mouth water and reignite her interest in eating. Tomato soup from a Heinz tin (she could tell if it wasn't) would remind her of our early trips, when Raj and I were children, to Srinagar in Jammu, Kashmir, to see her uncle who had been a high-ranking lieutenant general in the Indian Army. The tastes and smells never left her and with them came lost memories for her to experience afresh once more.

One of the summers we had together was a particular scorcher, which we were largely experiencing through the big windows of her room, and we were struggling to get Mum to take in enough fluid. Because her lucidity was always connected to hydration, Mum's water intake was always something we were massively aware of. As she loved sour things, I'd buy her lemon ice lollies or bring her iced water with fresh lemons and limes and tell her it was like Indian nimbu pani (lemonade). 'You'll like this one, Mummy,' I'd say, and she would drink happily.

I remember there was an advert that kept coming on TV during this baking-hot summer with a pile of berries on a plate. Each time this ad came into her field of vision she got really excited about it. She was such a creature of habit and routine she would never have bought that kind of thing in a shop, but now I went out and bought all these berries and made the plate up for her just like the one she exclaimed over on the TV.

It felt like an extraordinary moment when I served up all these ripe, plump strawberries mixed with deep red and purple berries with juicy pineapple and mango squares on a plate in front of her. It was wonderful to hear her coo and go, **'Ooo look at that, and for breakfast!'** The TV had always served as a reality check for her, and with those berries she understood the connection between different time periods. I found a huge amount of validation through the food I prepared for her and I felt I was making a meaningful difference to the quality of her life and her wellbeing. Seeing her eating food, having her favourite ice lollies, and enjoying drinking nimbu pani instead of tea, also nurtured and supported me.

I was already really practical when it came to what Mum needed. From the district nurses I learnt that Mum was eligible for some mobility aids that could help her. Handymen came as part of the package to install handlebars in the house and bathroom in order to help with Mum's mobility – she absolutely kicked off at this because she didn't want her interior décor ruined by these *not-so-stylish* mobility aids. In front of them, it was all smiles and 'thank yous', but to us she would vehemently say she **'didn't need them'**. But I knew she needed help between rooms and up and down the stairs to keep her safe. She even got a new mattress. **'What's wrong with the old one?!'** she railed at my sister who was on Mum Care during that outrage and had to deal with the fallout.

I also learnt to deal with what is probably the biggest taboo in caring for someone with a stoma and with dementia, but which was probably the hardest thing emotionally for Mum to cope with, and which must have hurt her pride indescribably.

The Gulati family were raised with impeccable standards of hygiene as well as a strong sense of shame around our bodies. I can remember as a little tomboy sitting with my legs akimbo and Mum getting mad at me and saying, **'Close your legs, Shobna, everyone can see your ham and bacon.'** Even in her decline, she could be uncomfortable around any suggestion of nudity.

I recall her being absolutely scandalized that I was wearing some leggings in a fleshy tone. It was one Christmas, when I had been rushing with a crazy work schedule and preparing Christmas dinner for everybody. **'What are you wearing, Shobi?**

I don't like it!' She spent the whole day telling me that I needed to go upstairs and put some clothes on, because she thought I looked too exposed. I hadn't brought anything else with me as I had dashed up the motorway, but she continued to be cross with me.

But I was used to it. This had always been an issue for her, not that she would have ever let anyone else comment on the racy pictures of me in the papers that she had so diligently collected, but when it came to the way I dressed at home she always had a problem. It all went back to the **'shame shame'** we were all brought up with regarding our naked bodies, and this loaded on the pressure around bathroom issues.

She had always been obsessively focused on her cleanliness to a meticulous level and us kids were always purged of any dirt. **'Have you washed your hands with soap?'** she would say every time we came in from outside. We even had 'outside' clothes, and she would get really cross if we didn't change straight out of our 'dirty' uniforms when we got home from school into clean home clothes. We had a rota for washing our hair – us girls could never wash our hair on a Thursday night because that was 'boys' day'; washing our hair would have been a sign of disrespect. Who knows where that came from? Plus Mum had a lifelong fixation with brushing our hair. If we wanted to soak in a bath, we had to have a shower first, so we didn't dirty the water; we weren't allowed to eat our breakfast before we had bathed or brushed our teeth.

Of course, cleanliness was a control issue for Mum, too. Cleanliness was essential and made up a huge part of our routine and traditions. Initially, Mum was really good at her stoma which was left after she recovered from bowel cancer. But then she wasn't, thanks to dementia.

Fairly early on, in either 2014 or 2015, Mum had gone to the bathroom when I realized that her stoma bag had leaked onto the floor of her room. I sat there, in front of the TV, absolutely frozen, not knowing what I should do. I suddenly thought, I've got to clean it up, but I also have to clean it up so she doesn't realize, as she'll go completely mad if she sees it. Or she'd be completely embarrassed. I didn't want to see either emotion – I just wanted to protect her. At the time I didn't even consider why she didn't know it was leaking, I was just entirely focused on hiding it from her. This was years before her diagnosis, after all. Luckily Sushma had secretly stocked the kitchen cupboards with loads of cleaning wipes – Mum would have gone on a tirade about it if she'd known, because she hated anything disposable. In that moment, I have never been so happy to see a single-use household product.

Later, as her memory faltered more, she'd forget about her stoma more frequently. But sometimes she'd also look at it and say wistfully, **'Raj says I can't have this reversed because I'm not well enough'** – even though it was her own doctors who had confirmed that she wouldn't be well enough for the operation, not Raj.

Sometimes, the biggest problem was often that she would point-blank refuse to go to the bathroom. Or she'd remove the bag in the night and forget to put another one on. Or we'd be sitting watching her soaps and I'd see that her stoma had been active and her bag needed emptying. I'd say, 'Mum, I think you need to go to the bathroom now.' She'd be like, **'Yeah, yeah, I'm just watching this – just let me go to the adverts.'** Then the adverts would come and go, and she still wouldn't move, so I'd say, 'Please, Mum, please.' What do you do in that situation? How do you manage a grown woman who really doesn't want to do something, and who has no notion of what is happening? Do you physically pick her up and take her to a bathroom? Or do you let her sit there and sit there and sit there, and hope she finally decides to go? When it's leaking everywhere, what do you do? Where is the advice on that?

Caring for your mother is not the same as when you care for
a child, when you just take them in hand and do what you know
is best for them. This is your mother, a woman who has been in
control of everything for your whole life and, what's more, she
doesn't even know what is happening. Or else she knows what's
happening but doesn't want to do anything about it. What can you
do at that point? I just used to take myself out of the room, take
some deep breaths and then slowly edge back in and do my best
to gently encourage her to the toilet. We'd go a few rounds, with
Mum saying, **'What do you think? That I don't know what I'm
doing? I don't need you.'** I'd oscillate between saying, 'No Mum,
you don't know what you're doing' and 'Of course you know what
you are doing, I'm here to help.' I'd try and be as gentle as possible
and not panic. That was usually enough to motivate her.

It was hard to work out the psychology you had to apply
sometimes, because there would be so many different versions
of Mum. She could be remembering and behaving like a child,
as a young woman, as my mother, as the widowed wife who had
been so capable, or as the lost mum who had forgotten where she
was in that moment. You never knew which one you would be
going toe to toe against. Would it be the belligerent mum? Or the
vulnerable, sweet child? Would it be the more lucid mum who
did actually know what was going on? Or would it be someone
entirely new? Should I be firm and strict? Did I have to make her
feel like I believed she was incapable to get her to do what was
best for her? It was a constant mental fight with yourself.

Sometimes there was just nothing I could do to prevent
accidents. It just became a part of the care. It was never about the
practicalities of the accident – you just tried to get on with the
cleaning or the sheet washing or bedclothes washing. But on a
deeper level it was the feeling that somehow you were taking away

her dignity which hurt, and you would do anything you possibly could to make her believe that *she* was keeping things together, that she 'didn't really need' our help. This worked for secret hoovering and night-time ironing and setting out her clothes, but it was harder when what I had to do was so personal and intimate, when I had to intervene at *that* point. I was trying so hard to protect her at all times, and it was really, really hard.

I had never seen her naked, she had always been so private and had concealed herself so carefully. I'd only ever seen her in her vest and bra when we went on that trip to India and shared a bed. This was my parent who had looked after me, an adult who had very strong opinions around nudity, shame and hygiene. The mother who wiped my bum when I was a small child and taught me how to 'toilet' and clean.

All of these things came into sharp focus when the two of us stood in the bathroom and Mum saw herself in the mirror, without her clothes on, her stoma excreting faeces. This was the worst of her worst-case scenarios. I would be on the floor trying to clean around her and she would scream at me, **'Get out. Get out of the bathroom. Don't touch it, you idiot, it's dirty. I know what I'm doing, you idiot. Get out!'** Her hand would hover above my head as I tried to pacify, clean and replace her bag quickly and efficiently. It was so painful to watch her, confused about why I was there, confused about what her stoma did and how it saved her life. And on top of the confusion there would be the fury at the shame she was being exposed to. I was exposing her simply by being there.

The only thing I could do was to help her in the moment, despite everything that was going on for her. The next day could come and she'd be different again and she might know exactly what was going on and be able to manage it all perfectly. The unpredictability of which Asha I was going to say good morning to took a huge toll on me emotionally. Some days brought relief, but others brought hardship.

Another one of the progressions of her disease was that Mum stopped getting changed out of her pyjamas if she wasn't 'going out anywhere'. She wasn't wearing her daily trousers and nice tops or salwar kameez any more, that fell by the wayside. On a Sunday before the havan (the religious service she attended with my brother), I'd lay out clothes on Mum's bed. After she'd showered she'd start worrying about what she was going to wear, and I'd lie and say, 'Well Mum, you've set it all out on your bed already, so I think you have already decided, don't worry about that.' Some days, even if we were expecting visitors, when I'd ask her to get dressed she'd say, **'So what, I'm just here and this is me.'**

Mum also stopped wanting to shower. Every day she was getting more and more tired and removed from keeping on keeping on, but every time she had to go out for an appointment or if we went anywhere, I coaxed her upstairs to wash herself. I didn't look forward to morning hospital appointments as this meant waking her up so early in order to start the gentle negotiation of what she was doing, where she was going, who she was seeing, the 'Shall we go upstairs to get ready?' and the repetition of it all without getting frustrated by it.

Some days she would brush her hair and other days not. Sometimes I'd ask if she wanted to go to the hairdressers and she'd say yes for a root colour and cut. Then she'd say no. But her desire to groom became rarer, and it got to a point that she never asked for it. I didn't give up because I knew she would feel better if she got spruced up. Some days I would spring a surprise visit, and after much coaxing we'd be sitting with Janet, her local hairdresser, by 3.30pm. Mum would always feel better when she got home. She recognized herself in the reflection. This mattered, so I never gave up.

Life became punctuated by rare but beautiful moments of tenderness between us, and moments of closeness that we had never experienced in our life together before. They would appear one day totally whole and beautifully painted, like a butterfly that only lives for a day. But they fluttered in and out of the house and made the tension, shame and loneliness all seem worth it. Even if they were only temporary, the sight and memory of them kept me going.

I introduced a different way of us being together after years of keeping our distance. Because of all her medication, Mum would often have headaches and I would massage her head and she just loved that. I'd rub moisturizer into her legs and did as much touch therapy as I could. I would massage her back and shoulders, even through her clothes. That kind of physical intimacy hadn't been part of our lives, I would never have touched her like that before, but I knew it was easing her discomfort and quietening her whirling mind. I'd sit up with her on her bed by the radiator and just be close, I even started kissing her forehead, she'd look at me as if to question it, but her eyes were full of the love and comfort it gave. Or sometimes she'd recognize that I might be tired, and would say, '**You can lie on my bed,** *beta,* **and take rest,**' then plump up the cushions for me.

Every day was different, and every day would also have its hard moments. Sometimes, every single minute of the day was different. But you would still see glimmers of the woman I had lost in among the new women who had begun to take her place, and the disquiet of the woman with dementia.

One day in September 2019 we were watching the news, and

there was this story about a gold toilet that went missing from Blenheim Palace. That really tickled Mum. **'Was it the Queen's toilet?'** she asked in fits of giggles. **'Where will the Queen go now her toilet is missing?'** she said starting to silently shake. **'Shobna, do you think her wee is so special it can turn another toilet gold?'** I burst out laughing at this farcical conversation. **'Loo larceny'** was what she called it. And as soon as it happened it was over and we were off somewhere else. She loved watching a repeat of *Top Gear, India*. Every time, she used to say the same thing, **'Who do these men think they are? They know nothing about India.'** Even in her decline she could still get fiery about being patronized.

Even through all of this she still refused to believe that she had dementia. If anyone mentioned the word in earshot, she would angrily snap, **'I haven't got that.'** Even when I tried to explain, your heart is ill, your kidneys are not well and your brain is poorly too, she would just not accept it. Sometimes she'd say, **'I don't know where my memory has gone to, I've forgotten what I was saying,'** and she'd laugh over an anecdote she couldn't recall any of the details of.

I stopped thinking about the future at all. I was too enmeshed in the duty of daily care and the world Mum now lived in, where her entire life was a great web we existed in, all hanging by a thread but in balance. There was a network of her mind that I didn't understand and nor did she, but it was connected, and although she couldn't choose which parts of her memory she would be shown or when she would be transported to them and nor could I, we were there together in among them.

So, we sat there side by side, cup of tea by cup of tea, breakfast, tablets, lunch, snack time, dinner, drink of water or no drink of water, loo visit by loo visit, from one moment of clarity to an angry outburst, to a near disaster to laughter which left us both silently shaking. Her recollections of her glamorous social life in stunning saris, arm in arm with my father, were now replaced by her memories of being a schoolgirl. We found our intimacy in it all, as we rowed out together into the unknown of her illness, never knowing what wave could crash into us next. But for now, we had one another, and we had those butterfly moments too. I just lived one wave at a time, one problem at a time, one small triumph at a time, one meal at a time, and sometimes I found myself quite lulled by the dependability of the routine and other times shocked by what the next day presented to me.

Sushma said to me, '**Let's get Mum to 80.**' And because, like a cat, she had nine lives – a stroke, a heart bypass, congestive heart disease, bowel cancer, dementia – it didn't seem implausible. I didn't see any end. I suppose I didn't want to see the end either. Despite all the rocks and the rapids, we were there together.

We just kept rowing out.

CHAPTER EIGHT

What's wrong with me?

Throughout the hot, sticky summer of 2019, I'd be by my mother's side from the moment she woke up. The fierce heat of the day found its way through the shut windows of her room. I had to open the windows in the kitchen and bathroom upstairs just to get some breeze through the house. But although it was stiflingly hot, Mum 'felt cold'.

Her health at this point was incredibly complex. The doctors were trying to medicate all her different illnesses, but each tablet had side effects, which meant she needed new pills to treat newly created conditions. Throughout the day she had to keep swallowing new colours, different sizes and different dosages of pills. We had to go through every new tablet and explain it thoroughly before she agreed to take it. It was a painstaking process – the medicine tightrope we'd been trying to carefully tread was becoming more and more precarious. Gone were the long periods where we were winning the fight. We were on a drastic rollercoaster dealing with her health issues.

She had recently been diagnosed with renal failure and hadn't wanted the rigmarole and commitment of dialysis. This was on top of her congestive heart disease and dealing with her stoma. Her dementia meant the dam we'd worked so hard to fortify for years was really starting to burst.

Every two weeks or so her kidneys packed up, sometimes they were overloaded with potassium, so then we had to change her pills and her diet all over again – and that would often have a knock-on impact on her overall wellbeing. It felt as though we couldn't solve one problem without creating another, more severe one. We looked endlessly for things we could feed her to help one of her issues, and then were terrified that we may have got it wrong. I remember Sushma in near hysterics because she'd given Mum a curry made with half a tin of tomatoes – they contain relatively low potassium levels in the scheme of things, but we were all on edge and hypervigilant. We looked everything up on the internet, investigated every minuscule ingredient for anything that might threaten her fragile equilibrium. But this was, in turn, futile, as she no longer wanted to eat anything, or drink anything for that matter. I spent a lot of time thinking, How can I get Mum to eat?

As soon as mealtimes approached, Mum was adamant that she'd already eaten – she'd forcefully inform us that she had just finished off a delicious plate of leftovers which she had reheated herself (of course), or that she had just had her breakfast moments ago, and couldn't be tempted by another meal, as she was too full. The sad irony was that when I was younger she made me eat every last morsel from my plate: how desperate I felt now the tables were turned.

Breakfast was always her ritual. **'You have to start the day right,'** she'd say, and she actually took her medication. By lunchtime I'd have to tell her she hadn't eaten again since breakfast. This would make her extremely frustrated, because her memory of eating and the passage of time was completely real to her, if false to us. She often told us that she felt sick and she'd only be comforted by the sour taste of fresh lemons with a little salt. I'd try to slice the lemons with deft precision, so as to make everything as appetizing as possible. It was really difficult to do anything more to make her better, while not destroying her perception of her wellbeing. We didn't want to unbalance what she felt was her grip on reality – it was real and true to her, even though it bore no semblance to the world in front of our eyes.

How a morning appeared to us was not how she saw it. Routine organized our days, but she had drifted far away from these constructs a long time ago, and trying to keep to a structure was like building a tower on ever-shifting sands. When it got to evening, I often couldn't find the motivation to cook yet another plate that would again remain untouched. Day in, day out, it had begun to wear me down. She was so vulnerable and I was so responsible for her, the woman who we wanted to keep in our world.

One night in October, exhausted by the effort of trying to tether her to reality, I thought, 'Let's just pick up a takeaway.' Takeaways or eating in a restaurant were always Dad's thing – we ate out together as a family every Sunday. It was a mega treat. Sundays were the day of the week we all looked forward to – it was Dad's only day off, in between working a five-day week plus his precious golfing on Saturdays – so we spent it together every single week.

We often went to watch Bollywood movies which were incongruously (and hilariously, in retrospect) screened at a soft porn cinema in Manchester city centre. Can you imagine it? This Indian family of six in their 1970s garb, speeding through the lobby of a somewhat suspect cinema, my mum with her hands over her little son's eyes as we got our tickets. I can remember her telling all of us to avert our eyes from the steamy posters you'd see as we walked in. I'd always sit next to Mum (on the other side was my brother) and, throughout the whole film, I'd whisper to her, 'What did he say? What just happened?', because my Hindi was just not that brilliant. It would drive her mad. **'Shut up, Shobna, I'm trying to watch. I'll tell you later,'** she'd hiss back, worried she would miss a critical bit in the story.

The Cameo cinema was just over the way from the Odeon, and right next door there was a Greek restaurant. I remember how much my mum loved avgolemono, Greek lemon, rice and egg soup. But Dad was always most fond of Chinese food and would teach us all the ways of chopsticks. He had his favourites on the menu and would always order: chicken and sweetcorn soup, egg fried rice, salt and pepper ribs, the sweet and sour fish, pork or chicken and various steamed dim sum treats, including chicken cashew, prawns and vegetables. My siblings and my parents would be in fits of giggles at my antics during these meals out at my turning my can of lemonade upside down in my glass and wiggling it around. I was being absolutely serious though – just like Mum I would be making sure I did not waste anything and got 'the last drop' out of the can.

So, to try and tempt Mum's appetite back that October evening, I decided on driving to a local Chinese restaurant, one Mum and I and the family had often frequented. By this point the car confrontations were well and truly over. Her car keys were left hanging on her elephant trunk hook without ever being disturbed. She'd just given up, or most likely forgotten about it.

It was another hostility that dissolved as she became much more sedate and calm. The keys seemed to serve as a talisman of parts of her we had already lost to dementia. Hanging there waiting to be used, yet never to be used again.

As I was about to set off, she asked to come along with me in the car. This was strange in itself, as she usually preferred to stay at home if I was only going to be a few minutes. When we got to the restaurant, I realized there were steps up to the door and no lift, so I had to leave Mum in the car. I wondered how quickly I could run in while keeping my eyes locked on her at the same time. I didn't ever want to let her out of my sight or for her to feel confused or abandoned. That said, I didn't know whether she'd even notice my absence. I opened the window a crack and said, 'Mum, I'll be back in a second,' then made the dash, tripping over my own feet on the way. I remember making it back to the car and feeling so relieved that she seemed safe and not distressed, while at the same time asking myself, What the hell was I thinking? Why have I ordered so much food for me and someone who doesn't eat?

I buckled my seatbelt and began to pull out, when out of nowhere she mentioned my dad. It was a visual prompt that had resurrected him in her mind – she had glanced out of the window and seen Royton Assembly Hall, which had been the venue of Mum and Dad's 25th wedding anniversary celebrations. Mum asked, **'Is it still a hall, Shobna? Do you remember? Your daddy used to bring me here.'**

It had been nearly three years since she'd spoken a word about him to me. The man who had meant everything to her, who she had built her identity around, had disappeared from her mind and memory until this very moment. I was struck dumb.

Every year our family would remember Dad's birthday and mark his death day, he was always in our thoughts. Before 2017,

Mum seemed present in those conversations, but something switched around the time she was diagnosed, and he vanished. Before that time, whenever she saw a handsome man, or as she talked to a young doctor, or mentioned her favourite movie star Rock Hudson, she would have a twinkle in her eye and say how Dad had been the only one for her. I remember her distinctly saying to me, **'If I had my time again, I'd marry your dad,'** even though, of course, by this point she had been without him for longer than they were together.

I started to scan back...and realized I couldn't remember when she had last mentioned him. Even before she stopped talking about him, she had always appeared quite matter of fact about my dad. Of course, none of us can see what happens within the layers of the mind, perhaps she did privately pine for him, but we spent enough time together over the years for me to believe she had found a way to cherish him but not long for him. The memory of him was fond and warm, she was not unhappy in her current situation and, dementia or no dementia, I think the milestone of remembering her silver wedding was significant, but not all together sad.

I will always remember my parents as being very much in love. Dad would hilariously shout, 'Mamaaa,' if he was stressed about having misplaced something. How she knew what he was shouting about always amused me, but she would just know – they were inextricably linked. Recently I have discovered a collection of cards they had sent each other. They had sweet nicknames for one another – *'Pochu'* for Mum, or 'my darling' for either of them – or else they simply called each other 'Mummy' and 'Daddy'. Far more affection could be said through the written word than could be spoken out loud. The letters are filled with love, indeed I was surprised to find how intimate with each other they were.

I suppose they had been very well trained in correspondence, living so much of their lives apart from their families on the other side of the world. It feels like letters have defined their story in a way that would be unfamiliar for young families today, we're so connected by the face-to-face zoom of fibre optics. Even as her mental capacity was in freefall, Mum still received cards from friends and family, both from home and abroad, and read them in full. Sometimes she would get confused over who had married, who had died, who had been born. Sometimes she would need our help and sometimes she surprised me with what she remembered. Like on that mundane drive to the fancy Chinese restaurant to pick up the takeaway.

'Do you remember? Your daddy used to bring me here.'

Everything seemed so upside down. It made me want to cry, but I held back my tears. It was usually me who asked the question, 'Do you remember, Mum?' – trying to force her mind to pick up the dropped stiches of her life. But that evening in the car, she asked me if *I* remembered.

My head spun as I replied, 'Of course I do Mum.' And we began to talk about the night of the party. As the conversation progressed, I noticed a strange shift in her approach, as if she suddenly believed she was talking to Dad and not to me. It was as if they were right back in the days when they were a very much in-love couple, and we would all go out to have his favourite Chinese food. I could see she was lost in that moment in time, and she was incredibly animated in a way that she hadn't been for so long. We drove back home and she ate a tiny bit of fried rice and 'seaweed', and that was Dad's interlude back into her life.

As I went to sleep that night, I thought about how dementia put every moment totally in flux, and sometimes what was lost could come back in the most surprising of ways. You just couldn't predict what would fall into her field of vision on any given day. In contrast to the earlier years of her illness, where adventures of her past life spilled into her present, new stories scarcely appeared through the haze now. And I was no longer let into the hidden parts of her life. The cogs of her mind had slowly but surely ground to a halt, as her physical needs became increasingly demanding and her memory contracted ever further.

Indeed, I did not know it then, but we would never talk about my dad again. That evening was his final curtain call.

As Mum's disease blunted the edges of her forcefulness, it also brought out a new, unexpected tactility.

One of the less pleasant things about spending a lot of time with an aging parent is that your social life starts to revolve not around celebrations but around funerals. A lot of the times we left the house together over these years were to attend a funeral of someone she had held dear. Often, she would forget they were dead and continue to speak of them in the present tense, but sometimes actually being there at their service helped her to understand that they had shifted out of the world we inhabited. She would share memories of her past, such as when Aunty Lilian died, and again we would be enveloped in the repeated comfort of the stories of her mum and dad's early years in England with Aunty Lilian when Mum was a baby. There was certainly an anxiety around people who were dead especially when she couldn't remember that they had died. She would murmur to me, **'Have they died?'** and I'd calmly tell her that, yes, they had, but you could see the confusion and the sadness at the loss replaying time and again. Mum was always very confused and distressed about Princess Diana, whom she had always loved, as she couldn't hold on to the fact she wasn't here any more. Any anniversaries or television coverage of her death would trigger a fresh wave of grief and upset.

On one occasion, however, it was Mum who accompanied me to the funeral of one of my friends, who had passed away at just 50. He had been one of my best friends when we were tiny, and I'd always seen him as a kindred spirit, because he didn't follow the rules of our strict Indian ways. As we arrived and took our seats, I was overcome with emotion. The weight of everything that was going on with Mum and the daily grind of caring for her were always conflated with any other kind of sadness, loss or hurt. It was as though I was already at full capacity, and if anything else was added on top of the load I was carrying I just couldn't find the strength to keep going.

But as I bowed my head and my eyes became overwhelmed with tears, my mother gently took my hand in hers and held it throughout the service. Perhaps she saw me as that little girl again. Perhaps it was because she had known my friend since we were children, or because she sensed I needed the support and her boundaries had been worn away.

When had she last held my hand that way?

When we had walked hand in hand away from the abortion clinic in 1994. Usually our family didn't need or expect physical affection. Or vocal affection either, really. We were all very self-sufficient in that way. Of course, if it was a question of safety when we were children, Mum held my hand to cross the road. It wasn't the contact itself which felt like a taboo between us, it was more that your hand would not often be held. I'm not like that as a mother either – I don't hug my son enough and sometimes he has to ask me to. That I have to make an effort to be physically affectionate is just the way I've been brought up. We kept things in, it wasn't in our nature to reach out and touch each other.

I think that's why Mum always liked speaking to us in the car, because no physical contact was required. She couldn't touch me even if she had wanted to and I think that made it easier for both of us to be truthful and more open about our emotions with one another. It almost made it a safe space. You couldn't really have a fight in the car, could you? Though when my dad was alive, he'd give it a fair go.

My friend who passed away was gay. He was just a tiny bit older than me, and in that time and that place, with our shared cultural background, to be homosexual meant there was a lot to fight. We wrote letters to each other when we were younger, and when Dad died there was some really intense correspondence between us. He had left the north for the bright lights of London, or 'Sin city', as we codenamed it. I had remained in Manchester. People in the community thought we were dating – being gay was so unimaginable – but of course we weren't, we just connected as kindred souls. When the community eventually found out, his treatment wasn't like that of the girls who had been disowned, the ones who would suddenly just disappear from family parties because their parents had cast them out. A gay man was unthinkable. They just ignored it because they couldn't get their heads around it.

Still, the most surprising thing about my mum holding my hand at his funeral was that she held it because I was distressed. I wasn't audibly crying, but she could sense my pain that day. She knew I needed the support of her holding my hand to get me through saying goodbye to that young man I had once been so close to. She had remembered.

Her old habits had started to fall away. Before 2017 she had always been impeccable with her presentation. What I'd always found extraordinary about her was how little she sought validation, not from men, not from anyone. She dressed for herself, she coordinated her lipstick to her sari for her own pleasure and she wore jewellery simply because she loved to be beautiful for her own eyes. But by this point even her pyjamas didn't match, and she didn't even notice or rather she didn't care.

Yet some things were encoded in her so deeply that they never lost their power over her. Right to the last, she didn't want our help in the bathroom, even when she really needed it. She also never failed to wash her hands, and if you came into the house she would always ask if you'd washed yours too. You had to do that before anything. If she was sitting in front of the telly with some jammy toast, the minute she finished she'd mention her tacky hands and then keep reminding herself that she had to wash them – but these days she never made it to the sink, there was always something on the TV distracting her, so she would hold out her hands in front of her so she wouldn't touch anything. (I would get a wet wipe and say, 'I'll do this for now, then you can wash them later.') Her household would always remain a place where sticky doorknobs, sticky surfaces or fingers were verboten.

She had always had milk delivered by the milkman and she used to be very particular about it – even the milkman had to follow her ways. To ensure that birds weren't attracted to the shiny tops, she left out two empty, cleaned-out yoghurt pots and asked the milkman to put them over the bottles like lids. Even though she switched to drinking skimmed milk, she still thought the birds would get the cream. Waking up and bringing the milk in had been a key part of her morning routine. The funny thing was, she wouldn't forget to tell you to put out clean yoghurt pots the night before, but she would forget to collect the milk in the morning. If I'd been away, I'd sometimes arrive home to off milk on the doorstep, or the morning would roll around to 10am and

I'd realize we didn't have fresh milk in the fridge. **'Oh yes, I was going to get it,'** she'd say. So eventually we stopped the milk round and we bought it from the supermarket instead, and none of those bottles needed guarding from potentially thirsty birds. Such was my acceptance of these micro-changes that it never struck me as sad that something like getting the milk in, which she had fiercely protected for so many years, could slip away from her day-to-day existence so easily.

Although she never forgot the yoghurt pots or to clean her hands, the number of things that did slip away exceeded those that didn't. Whenever you left Mum's house, she'd always come to the door to see you off. She'd wave you out of her drive, **'Call me when you get home'** even if your home was just down the road. It was my favourite thing – I called it the **'OK, bye, OK, bye'**. Mum would stay on the doorstep and wave constantly until you had truly left. When we all lived there as a family, we were often under instruction to show guests out this way. In Mum's mind it was polite and gracious, but I found it quaint and funny. Sometimes it took ages and I always felt we were putting our visitors under pressure to just *go!* As her health deteriorated, however, Mum started to send me to the door to do the **'OK, bye'**. And then even that habit of making sure someone saw the guest off stopped too. Just on one random day, and it never came back.

Those small parts of her that I'd taken for granted kept disappearing without ceremony. I never really knew the exact point when they left, but one day I would realize that they had gone in a puff of smoke, as if they had never really happened in the first place.

It was also around this point that it became impossible to settle her. Anyone caring for a person with dementia will recognize this struggle and will have experienced moments when their

constant feeling of unease becomes overwhelming. I would notice
she was becoming antsy and it would soon escalate to becoming
impossible to get her to sit. It wasn't as though she could really
walk around anywhere, it was more that she would constantly

lie down,

get up,

lie down,

get up,

say, **'I've got a headache'**,

say, **'I've not got a headache'**,

say, **'I don't feel well'**,

say, **'I'm fine'**,

say, **'I don't feel sick'**,

say, **'I feel sick'**,

say, **'I just can't settle'**,

Then forget what she had said.

She didn't want to be in her bed,

she didn't want to sit against her cushions on her bed,

she also didn't know where else she would like to be.

These periods would make my heart ache. It felt like I was in a
battle. I would try everything in my arsenal – iced drinks, food, TV,
cards, jokes – to soothe her both physically and mentally. When
nothing worked, I'd pull out the photo albums to try and prompt
her memory, to transport her to a time or a place outside the
current one. But this too had stopped working.

As for the world outside, it had evanesced like a sun-bleached
photograph. Keeping up with all the politicians' names was
beyond Mum, but she could recognize Boris Johnson when he
came onto the TV, from when he was Mayor of London, and
she would comment that she didn't like his hair. **'Look at this**

namoona...' (look at this 'specimen' of a human) with deep sarcasm. The same language was used for Nigel Farage.

Dementia doesn't change your perception of a fool nor your prerogative to cast your ballot, and you are allowed to bring along a helper as long as they are a close relative. I helped Mum vote twice and I found that difficult – there is something about the sanctity of a private vote that runs so deep in our psyche. As she had always leafleted and campaigned, and had been a participatory person her whole life, there was no way we were going to let her voice go unheard. We had conversations before election days and made sure we tuned into the news to try and help her to have the best understanding of what was going on. Mum was proud to vote Remain in the EU referendum, reminding us she had voted previously for the Common Market. When it came to the general election in June 2017, I went into the booth with her and read out all the candidates' names, telling her which one was associated with each party. To her, to exercise her franchise was always something she considered to be of the utmost importance, and we all respected that.

As we moved into the longer dog days of the summer of 2019 she couldn't stay still, no matter what was on the TV. Any semblance of focus had dissipated. These days I couldn't leave her side without her crying out that she needed me for something or other. I had to do all the food shopping when she was sleeping, and I'd dash back because I would be in an absolute panic that if she woke up and I wasn't there she would become very distressed.

I had become very anxious too. My life had been on hold for years; now the cord with anything to do with my own existence was cut. I made an exchange of my life for hers, because we wanted to give her the best quality of life for the years and months she had left. She wanted to be at home, so Team Mum

Care made sure we kept her there.

Looking back, I wonder if her attachment to home, 'Geetangali', was subconsciously something to do with Dad after all. He had had that house built for them, and when she was there, he was with her. I will never know, because she couldn't tell me. All we were ever told was, **'I like my house.'** And whenever she went away to stay with my siblings she would smile on her return. **'I'm so pleased to be home, put the kettle on.'**

I often turn my mind now to whether, if Mum hadn't been at home in her own environment, with us all around her every day, she would eventually have forgotten us completely. But because we were so involved in her life, so in her business, she couldn't let go of us. She'd cared for all the grandchildren and she knew the minutiae of the family dynamic and that meant we were constant reminders. Just across from her bed was a row of all their school photographs – her own rogues' gallery as she called it – so there was a constant visual cue. But it was almost as though we irritated her into remembering us. The family dramas, of which there were at least three raging at any one time, provided her own personal soap opera to watch over and over again. There was always something for her to talk about, or indeed complain about.

Whether it was me and my idiotic choices of boyfriends, or being an actress, or being in some story in the paper, or Sushma travelling up and down like a bungee, and whatever else was going on with her kids or her husband, or Raj and his wife and kids, or Hema and her husband and children, or Akshay and me, each storyline had enough plot to ensure she remained gripped by the family saga. After all, she truly was the woman at the centre of every drama; she was the leading star of this family soap opera: The Gulati Show.

CHAPTER NINE

Why are you feeding me?

And then she started slipping through my fingers. The fragments on to which we'd been holding so tightly, fluttered out of our grasp in bursts. The stoma accidents became the norm rather than the exception, her recollections yet more adrift. No more looking forward to breakfast, lunch or dinner. No more excitement about *Coronation Street*. No more changing the channel on the remote control to catch up on yet another repeat. No more quick wit. This mighty woman, my indomitable mother, dimmed darker and darker into the shadows.

As Mum's condition crumbled, caring for her began to demand every ounce of my love and devotion. It tested everything about me, my very core was stretched. The days started to break us all, though in some ways I felt that I had deeper reserves to dig into than ever before. Caring for my mum had changed me, adding resilience and stamina that I had never before recognized as part of myself.

Part of that was because I had found a new sense of acceptance of the kind of carer I had become. I had always felt that there was something inherently creative in the art of caring. I wish somebody had told me at the start that it was OK to do things in your own way – to bring your unique skills and personality to your time as a carer. It would have saved me a lot of second guessing myself, and guilt for not living up to what I thought she deserved. I'd always had this sense that a carer needed to be nurse-like and probably a bit more organized than me, detached but caring. I suppose that's what we see in the media. Of course, I had always taken advice from leaflets and had done my best to exercise Mum's memory, make sure she was well fed and watered, and had all her medication on time – to do all the things the doctors and healthcare workers suggested. We all followed the advice. But that only covered so much time; the rest of it, I eventually realized, was really down to you and your temperament.

For me that meant using my imagination. It was filling the house with delicious smells when she was feeling physically unwell in a bid to encourage her to eat. It was keeping her lucid and hydrated with lemony iced drinks. It was knowing the prompts and working with them to keep her engaged. There was even creativity in the way I obscured who was doing the housework and the stories I ad-libbed to make her feel a sense of dignity. I even became a stand-up comedian with my own self-deprecating routine to make her feel better about her appearance or how she was feeling. 'Don't worry, Mum, look at me – I've dragged myself through a hedge backwards this morning,' to which she'd answer, **'You must have had a fight in your sleep.'** Then I'd say, 'Yes, I look like a nightmare!' and she'd laugh, and we would manage to brush her hair.

I sort of made it up as I went along, but looking back my caring personality started with empathy, to identify her desires and needs, and finished with creativity, to problem-solve and help create security and joy for her. As soon as I realized that, I felt what you could describe as confidence in my role. And that made what lay ahead just that little easier to cope with.

Aside from being a creative carer, I also helped her break the rules. Sometimes, even in those days when despair was so close at hand, she would whisper to me, **'Can I have some sugar on these strawberries, Shobi?'** I knew Sushma, as a dentist, would kill me if I put too much sugar on, but I'd be naughty for Mum. But also safe – there was a sugar shaker that didn't shake out too much sugar, so that was a win-win in my book. Both Mum and Sushma would be OK. I enjoyed being impish, news that will surprise no one. I do think that's why we got on more often than not during this time, because I always remembered that she was my mum, and I wasn't hers, even if it was my job to take care of her. If she wanted to have her little rebellions in her own home, why not? She was entitled to it.

Every time Sushma came over she'd tell me off affectionately about the treacle toffee in Mum's snack cupboard. Mum absolutely loved those toffees. Packets of them. To be fair to Sushma, she'd always looked after Mum's teeth and she was really upset when Mum lost a tooth in a piece of toffee. Mum, as ever, saw the funny side, telling the tale of how she was dead-set on writing a letter of complaint to Thorntons about the outrage of finding a tooth in her toffee, before she realized it was actually hers.

I also really learnt to think on my feet when it came to explaining things to Mum that she had forgotten. I never wanted to say, 'Yes, I already told you, Mum,' when she failed to recall things, which now happened minute to minute. So, when she woke up on the morning of a doctor's appointment and hadn't the foggiest why I was chivvying her along, I'd come up with some madcap story about a last-minute appointment or a late-night call from Raj, so she wouldn't feel the weight of knowing she had forgotten something. It was like improv – all that acting training came in useful. I just used to think how wearing it would be if somebody was constantly saying to you, 'I told you, I've said that, do you remember?' Of course, I could never be sure what that would mean to her, but I often imagined how mad it would make me.

It wasn't like she always appreciated all my efforts and it's not like all the emotion was taken out of our relationship just because she had dementia. It's very difficult when you've taken the time and energy to do something special for someone and what you do for them is either rejected or ignored. I found that really hard and I think that's because I've craved validation from everyone, and especially my mum, my whole life. My mum wasn't ever one to beat about the bush – if she didn't like something you'd made or done for her, she would tell you. You would be the *namoona* (like Boris), or an *ullu* (stupid owl), also like Boris.

Ultimately, you just have to carry on. I had to try and not take it personally, though it did feel personal. You do become somewhat hardened to it over time, and I knew it wasn't just me who felt those occasional stomach punches. Sometimes, for a change of scenery, or because I needed support for work, I drove Mum down to Sushma's and she made this gorgeous cosy room up for her, with a TV just as she liked it, and all her things around her. But Mum would complain and wouldn't settle, she wanted to go home, and that was very demoralizing for Sushma and me.

There were lots of times that, no matter what, you didn't or couldn't satisfy her. Everything you did was met with consternation. It took me a long time to truly believe and accept this was no one's fault: not hers, not mine. I carried that feeling of not being up to the job for years. Making the mental separation and acknowledging that these situations are happening because of dementia, because of her condition as opposed to her feelings for you, was so important.

By the end of the summer of 2019, Mum was really struggling with the concept of time, night or day. She had an LED display clock next to the TV and we tried to help her keep a record of the hours going by – pointing to the date and asking her to match up the day on the clock with that on her tablet dosette box. When we'd ask her to read the display she would say, **'So late,'** then mischievously say, **'Why did you wake me up, it's too early, we've got so much time?'** Sometimes in the evenings, she'd be put out: **'Are you going to bed now, Shobi? It's only 10pm!'** The device was there for her to look at – she had the immediate thoughts of 'What's the time?' but then moved on without taking it in: time wasn't a tangible thing for her any more. Those dates and times on her calendar, once so important, were now just arbitrary.

She had never wanted to be rushed, nor had she ever been a morning person, but it became increasingly difficult to get Mum up. Her breathing was also an issue – it was becoming more and more laboured every day. We had an oxygen machine installed in the house, so I started to give her ten minutes of oxygen as part of our daily routine, especially if she had to go out, which was fairly frequently due to the countless hospital appointments needed to manage her conditions.

Since Raja was always the one to take her, the appointments

were scheduled for 9am so he could fit them around work. I can tell you, getting a woman with dementia up, washed and dressed and waiting at the door for 8.30am is like completing an assault course. I'd lie in bed and think, I'm just going to do it, I'm going to go in there and throw open the curtains and be as breezy as possible.

'Hi Mum!' I would boom, beaming at her and trying not to think about the battle ahead. **'No, no, no, no. Go away, I'm sleeping,'** would be the first response. So, I'd start talking about the *delicious* breakfast I'd made her and how lovely it was all going to be. I would explain where she was going in every which way I could, as she would ask me every minute or so. I used every ounce of my positivity to get her going. She would be full of rage, so I'd crack jokes and try and get her to smile. Finally, she would give in. By the time they left, I'd feel like I'd run the gauntlet.

Our family WhatsApps were full of reports of her mood, and as the leaves began to crisp and turn to russet, Mum's spirits began to darken. 'She's very prickly today' meant that you were in for a thankless day and there was very little you could do to improve her state of mind. As things sped downhill, finding the mental discipline not to beat yourself up about things was more important than ever. I continued to write poetry in the mornings while I waited for her to wake up. It really helped me to digest some of the feelings I was dealing with, as well as to work through a lot of the issues that had been plaguing me for years. In that sense, creativity saved me too.

Everything was hard. Every simple, single thing.

There was a new frailty to my mum. When she had a bad physical episode of ill health, she hardly moved out of her bed, or from sitting on the cushions on her bed, and her muscles atrophied.

Her communication also became fraught, her language more limited, and it felt as if, day by day, she was detaching herself from us. I thought that her brain, its cells perishing at an ever-increasing rate, was also beginning to distort her coordination and articulation. The atmosphere in her room had changed completely. She was often quiet. It was incredibly sad. We had very little idea of where she was retreating to because she couldn't tell us. I think she didn't even know herself.

Dementia is an incurable, progressive, relentless disease. It's not, 'Here, you've got a headache! Take some paracetamol.' Or even, 'It's cancer, let's try radiotherapy.' There's nothing you can do except make someone as comfortable as possible. It is impossible to imagine until you know by experiencing it how hopeless that can feel. There's a certain denial that takes place within you when someone is diagnosed with dementia and you just hope their experience isn't going to be a 'bad one'. Yet you know, if you're honest with yourself, that it's a life sentence. It is a terminal disease and it brings death nearer. Even if you can live with it for many years, it's not going to go away. I think we all expect death to be so dramatic, like something you see dramatized on TV or in films, but for someone with dementia it's a *process* of dying. There's no shocking moment, it's just a slow, inexorable, often painfully drawn-out procession towards the end. That's something that we all had to accept, and as siblings we managed it differently. Some of us reached a state of acceptance and slowly came to terms with what was staring us in the face, but for others it was harder to confront. All of us, however, exchanged years of our lives to care for Mum. That was the bargain we struck.

By September that pact was beginning to falter under the sheer, overwhelming strain. For the first time the question of care outside of the family was raised in earnest. Raj started the family's discussion, because Mum's increasing needs, especially with regard to the bathroom, were making things untenable. From my experience, my brother under stress is not the world's most patient person, and, for Mum, losing control in front of him was the very, very worst thing that she could have ever imagined. It wasn't an ideal dynamic for either of them and navigating her now significant issues with her stoma was bad news for all of us. He just said, 'I can't do it any more,' and I was tasked with looking into the options.

I think, looking back, that Raj was overwhelmed by how dementia was affecting her. When it came to Mum's physical health he'd done his very best to keep everything balanced, and he always seemed comfortable with that side of things, even having her over to his home to be with his family some weekends. Watching your parent suffer with dementia is brutal, and however 'educated' or medically knowledgeable you are, it is a very different thing to watch it take everything away from a person that you love. It has no logic, nor routine, nor precedent from person to person. It took years for me to understand that I could not control Mum's dementia or stop it from progressing. It wasn't anybody's fault. Team Mum Care had to forgive each other and ourselves individually for those times when we just couldn't cope.

I was due to begin work at the Lyric Theatre in Hammersmith for the panto season and rehearsals were starting in October with the run through November, December and the beginning of January. Twelve show weeks meant I was limited to how much I could take on. Raj's reticence to be more involved when I was away at work reduced our options. The only solution would be a care home, something we had discounted for so many years, so averse to it because it really wasn't an option in our community. Nor in our cultural DNA.

Even though we had a social worker assigned to Mum, it wasn't easy to assess the available pathways when you are new to the care system or to gauge what is good and what isn't. I was entirely at a loss to work out what would be best for her. We felt that with her particular needs Mum needed 24-hour nursing care, but I wanted to ensure that there would also be a consideration and understanding of Mum's heritage where she would be living.

I rang around trying to find care homes with residents or staff from our cultural background or with similar 'lived' experience to Mum's. I couldn't find any. I called around some of my friends and had a couple of places recommended to me, but nothing seemed appropriate.

Mum threw a spanner in the works from the get-go. When we got someone to assess her in order to see what level of nursing care she needed, she suddenly appeared much more lucid and responsive. I know it wasn't deliberate, I just think she wanted to present her best self to the new strangers in her house. But it was hugely frustrating – because of that assessment, we were told Mum was ineligible for nursing care and she would have to be put into a generic residential home for the elderly, which wasn't what we'd hoped for. We also all knew that Mum didn't want to go into a care home, but we were close to breaking. One day in mid-October, I went up to Manchester from London in the morning, down to London for a rehearsal, then back up to Manchester the same night. It had started gnawing at the edges of my sanity.

The pressure of everything led sadly to a crisis with my brother. As a carer you aren't offered any mental health support by the state, or even a route to deal with these kinds of family flare-ups, which are inevitable when things get really bad. All the issues over the past years with Mum, and of course the years preceding her condition, surfaced once again. Some very hurtful things were said that could never be taken back. Our social worker stepped in and suggested a couple of places that might work better for Mum, and after visiting them all – again, no mean feat when you literally have no time and are full of emotion – I found one which I thought might just be right. The room she would stay in was really lovely, and though I wasn't entirely sure about the communal space or front of house, I reserved a place for her and crossed my fingers.

Part of a care home's assessment involves an at-home visit and we all suspected that Mum would be pretty hostile, but by this stage we couldn't predict how she would behave from one moment to the next. She had become mercurial and even the most defined sides of her personality had shifted. When the women from the home came to visit Mum, they talked everything through with her very gently and, for a second, I thought she might have accepted that she needed help. The opposite was the case. She turned to me, staring directly into my eyes and said, **'Shobi, I do not want to go for a holiday, I do not want to go for a visit. I do not want to go to any kind of home. I want to stay here.'** There was no way of explaining to her *why* she would be going. She remained fixed on staying at home.

Mum's emotional reaction to the discussion around assisted living put us in an impossible situation. If my brother was going to drop his part in the care chain and I still needed to work to keep up any semblance of a career or financially viable life, I felt there were no good choices. But the guiding force had always been the need to make sure that Mum got what she wanted until she died, so emotionally, deep down, I knew we just had to make it work for her.

Sushma managed to get over to see the home and came back and said, 'You're right Shobi, the room is very nice…But I don't think it's the place for our Mum.' I knew she was right, but I was tearing my hair out trying to find a way forward. I decided that I was going to give up working entirely and called my agent to say I couldn't do it any more. It was at that moment that Sushma stepped in and told me that I had to carry on working. She offered to increase her days in the care rota and even suggested that we move Mum to her home in Hertford, so she could be closer to my work for us to share the hours, without either of us ping-ponging up and down the motorway. Raja said to Sushma, 'That's all I needed to know.' He was completely depleted.

But although this solution seemed viable, and Sushma meant it completely sincerely and from her heart, the reality of getting Mum set up with the assorted team of specialists she now needed to manage all of her different conditions felt like an impossible obstacle to overcome. It takes time for medics to get to know any situation, understandably, and we were really worried about starting that process all over again. Of course, it would have been *possible*, but as anyone who has worked within the NHS system will know, *possible* and *manageable* can often be entirely different things.

I was also aware that Mum knew her hospital, her environment, the stoma nurse, the district nurses, so intimately. We probably got a level of preferential treatment, for better or worse, because Mum was quite the personality, and also Raja worked at the hospital and Dad had too. The other point was that, yes, the geography would change and that would ease the logistics for us, but there would be the same frustrations of caring for Mum and her conditions, and they would come in Sushma's family home, meaning she would be unable to escape the very real pressures. Moving to Sushma's would not cure Mum. There was no cure. I knew it would put an enormous strain on Sushma's family life and that wasn't fair. So despite my sister really wanting to do it, I was really reluctant to usher in the changes.

So, for the rest of October, the plan was that I'd work in the morning and afternoon then dash up to Manchester on the night bus or train or in my car. I would coordinate between Sushma, Jayshri, Akshay, myself and Raj, if he could. I didn't have that many late-night finishes, just early-morning starts. By this point Sushma was working for herself, another development which helped us to understand each other's lives. We knew it was going to be tough, but I felt supported and closer than ever to my sister.

Then all at once everything completely fell apart. In the middle of the week, before I was due to leave for London for rehearsals all guns blazing, I called Raj to say that Mum seemed to be struggling more with her breathing. He came over as normal on Wednesday and said he thought she was OK, but on Thursday it had gotten a lot worse. When Raj arrived to check on Mum on the Friday, he said we needed to get her admitted to hospital.

That Saturday morning, I got Mum up and dressed early and we sat together on her bed, waiting for my brother to arrive. I remember being so heartsick getting her ready, knowing that I'd be so far away while she was in hospital, and she had no idea what was to come. It was always difficult to leave her when I went to work, no matter what, but this felt ominously different, as though she was going to have to face this next battle alone. None of us was going to be able to help her with this one, as this was a fight only she could take part in. As we sat side by side, Mum once again reached out and held my hand. I held back on my emotions and did my best to reassure her: 'You're just going into hospital because we just need to make sure your breathing steadies up.'

Every hour I was away that week, I thought about her. It was impossible to disentangle myself, no matter what was going on with Mum, and sometimes I thought I was losing it trying to be professional in my work life while going through all of this in the background. It was so hard to keep my focus on anything else except for the WhatsApp messages pouring in from my siblings and my son, who had travelled to be with his nani. Sushma told me she felt Mum was deteriorating quite rapidly, and she wasn't eating anything at all. By the time I arrived back at the end of the week, Mum had changed significantly. She was really, really distressed.

From being a woman for whom physical contact was something reserved exclusively for her husband or her son, Mum barely let go of our hands, gripping as tightly as she possibly could. She was completely locked into her anxiety. She didn't know where she was, or what she was doing there, and she was very frightened. Mum kept saying to me, **'Shobi, I'm scared, I'm scared. Am I dying, am I dying?'** Her head was constantly in pain and her mannerisms became very erratic and fraught. We couldn't settle her for even the space of a few minutes, she was up and down and up and down like a jack-in-the-box, and with the same spring of nervous energy. She had always been slow and methodical in everything that she did, but here in hospital it was like she was in a frenzy, as if she were trapped in a struggle. At night she ripped out all of her wires and tubes, the catheter and everything monitoring her, trying to escape. The weeks of rejecting food had taken their toll on her physicality, and without the layers of her cardigans she looked absolutely tiny. Looking at her, sitting there in her hospital gown, my every maternal instinct was triggered. It was like she was disappearing. Replacing our powerhouse of a mother was a very, very frightened little girl.

Our plan was to try and get Mum out of hospital as quickly as possible and into 24-hour care at a nursing home. It would be the best place, given the fragile situation between the members of Team Mum Care. She would be surrounded by nurses who would be able to understand where she was physically and mentally. In my head, they would be able to cope much better than us, and that would mean that Mum would be better. But, because she'd been assessed only a few weeks prior, when we had investigated assisted living, we were told she was ineligible for this type of nursing care, no matter how much her condition had worsened. Even though Mum's health had obviously failed significantly enough to require hospitalization, the previous assessment apparently stood.

It began to become clear to all of us, although unsaid, that Mum was out of her nine lives.

On my return, at the end of the second week, I'd brought an award that I'd just won – a big piece of glass with my name on it, exactly the kind of thing that Mum would have always liked. For a split second when I showed it to her she smiled at me and I saw a glimmer of her old self, but then her face contorted back into fretfulness and she was lost beneath its surface again.

There was something telling us that Mum just had to come home as soon as possible. She had been in hospital for nearly two weeks and she had become unrecognizable from the woman who had held my hand on the bed the week I started work. We came up with a plan with the help of our social worker and managed to put palliative care into her home. Raj replaced her bed in the living room with a nursing bed, and from London I called around to organize the different care teams through a hospice-at-home service.

On the Thursday, Raj phoned us all to let us know she was back home. I immediately stepped out of work, and as my train came into Manchester I realized my sister Hema's daughters were on board too – the whole family was about to fill the house which had for so many years just been Mum, me, her bed and the TV.

When I arrived, Mum was in the new bed, completely mute. She was very calm and was completely quiet, but she had stopped speaking. Occasionally she nodded and appeared to be listening to what was happening around her—Sushma, busy cleaning, trying to focus her grief into sorting the house ready for everybody's visit, my nieces in and out, chatting between themselves. My instant feeling was that I needed to try and get her to eat something, as it had been more than ten days since she'd managed anything. One of the clearest signs that a person suffering from dementia is nearing the end of their life is when they stop wanting to eat and drink. Their memory has become so poor that they can't recall what food is any more, it becomes a foreign body in their mouth. Oftentimes they can forget how to swallow and lose coordination of their mouth, but with Mum at the hospital it had just seemed a deep disinterest.

I started cooking in Mum's kitchen, as I had so many times before, thinking of all the things she'd have to say about how I was using her pans, spoons and the cooker and cutting her onions. I thought about all the times she would love to hate us 'overtaking' her things, with all of us in the house.

I knew that some of her senses might still be working, including her sense of smell, so I hoped the familiar scents of home cooking wafting through the hallway and into the downstairs rooms would serve to comfort her. In the past, when Hema and her family visited, there would always be a mountain of food to prepare, she'd often be stressed and I'd often help, as I really love cooking. Now, I wanted her to know I would have her back, and be able to cook food for everybody, and she would not have to worry about any of it. It was OK, I had it under control.

She could just 'relax'. All these sorts of thoughts were running through my mind and I just wanted to comfort her in the way I always had.

I cleared her room of Sushma, her son, her husband, Raj and my nieces, as I knew that Mum was more likely to eat if it were just the two of us. I needed some quiet with Mum so she could be with me, and I with her, totally. As I sat down with a plate of her favourite daal, plain boiled rice and natural yoghurt, she looked up at me. Until then, Mum had been dead silent, but after she ate a few spoonfuls, she quietly asked, **'Why are you feeding me?'** That question told me that she knew she was dying. She wasn't asking me to say, 'Why are you feeding me, you idiot, have you lost your mind?' or 'Why are you feeding me, I'm not useless, I can feed myself.' Instead, I think she asked me because she knew she was ready to go.

After she finished her small bowl, we sat together watching her television. Then everyone was back in the room, and an advert came on with someone taking their clothes off – her eyes widened at the man's nakedness, with that once ever-present 'faux' shock of mischievousness. As Sushma walked into the room, I said to Mum, 'Who's here?' and she replied, **'Sushma.'** We then watched a documentary on Prince Charles, who she recognized clearly, saying his name aloud: **'Prince Charles.'** All those Lady Di clippings that once lived under her old bed, now tidied away under the table in her room to make a proper space for her care, were obviously still deeply embedded in her mind. And those were the last words I heard her utter.

And so our rhythms had played out once again, smaller than they once were. I cooked and fed her, Sushma tidied and cleaned up, Raj was there to keep an eye on her condition. Those were our roles, ones which had been set years before.

With everyone in the house for the next two nights, and the palliative nursing teams coming and going, I decided to go home to sleep in my own bed. I knew that my mum might pass away in the night, but I also knew she was surrounded with love and, in some ways, I had started to let go.

When I returned to the house on the Saturday morning, I realized Hema's daughters had left. The atmosphere was so heavy you could hardly breathe. Everyone was coming close to grief and we knew that our uneasy alliance based on Mum's present need was coming to a close.

It had always been strained for us siblings, but I knew we had to keep it together for Mum. Sushma and Raj were at silent loggerheads as I walked in, so I knew I needed to say something. I calmly said, 'Look, Mum might have had a stroke, she might have dementia, she might be dying, but she can still feel. She can feel this atmosphere. Even someone with the latest stages of dementia can pick up on the distress of the people around them. Whatever is going on, we've got to calm this. *Now*.' Hema was due to arrive from India that evening and Akshay and Sushma's daughter, Nina, were driving up together that morning, so there were going to be even more personalities in the mix before we blinked. I knew that we needed to all sit down and make a promise to be there together for our mum. And we did. The three of us joined together and held hands and we quelled the storm.

The night before, I'd made the decision that I was going to say goodbye to Mum on Saturday. My big sister, Hema, was arriving in the evening; I didn't want to be there for her arrival and I didn't want Mum to pick up on the inevitable tension between us either. Hema and I had had our differences over the years, and they had come to a head during the difficult period of caring for Mum. Our relationship was over. But I had promised Mum to forgive our differences, so it felt like the right thing for my sister to have her chance to be with our mum. She'd not been a constant in Mum's life for so long because she lived in India. I felt Hema deserved that space and time with her, without our personal drama.

I'd been in and out of the trenches with Mum for years and we had come to an understanding. I knew where she was at in the end and we had said and done everything that we needed to. I understood that there were some difficult memories between Mum and me too, but we had made our peace. It is a human thing, we all can slip at own peril and sometimes we hurt ourselves and the people we love. For me it was never intentional, though the consequences have been huge. I feel so lucky that I had 25 years to get there with my mum; 25 years to redeem myself for what had happened. The wrapping of that gift is Akshay. If it hadn't been for him, I might never have had this time to get to know her. I had needed her and she had stepped up.

I don't think either Mum or I consciously decided to reconcile, it's just how it happened. We forgave each other for everything that we had done to each other and offered nothing but gratitude for the support and care we had shared during our moments of need, through both duty and love. We were always there for each other, my mum and me. It was the realization that my mum always had done the very best she could, that my parents always 'did what they thought was right'. I know she was OK with me in her final moments. That is all I could have hoped for.

Akshay would stay behind, able as ever to bring everyone together in a way I never could, so it felt like a part of me would still be there with her in him. I walked into Mum's little room holding a vanilla Mini Milk ice lolly, which I knew she would like more than anything else. She relished it as I fed her for the final time.

We said our goodbye.

It was incredibly painful and it was hard not to change my mind, but with a momentum borne from knowing that if I stopped for a second I wouldn't be able to keep on going, I threw my bag in the boot and started the car, driving south away from my family, as I had done so many times before, going to work.

That Sunday morning, I woke up in London alone just before 5.30am, feeling my heart hammering in my chest with the massive rush of cortisol pumping around my body. In the silence, in that waking moment, I just knew: she was gone.

A few minutes later, the phone went and Raj told me that she had died. Memories of hearing those early-hours phone calls. Memories of my mum taking those calls that informed her of the untimely deaths of her father, her husband and her mother. I was so overcome that, after speaking to my son, I descended away from the distressing reality and back into sleep.

When I woke up again, I felt a true sense of contentment. It was all so right. As I set off to work, my safe space, to record a BBC radio comedy series, of all things, I thought about the many times my life had been presented with similar juxtapositions. The countless times that I had managed to do what I needed to do when behind the scenes at home things were so far from being OK. The joy and happiness I'd managed to project as an actress and a dancer when everything in my real life had been strained to breaking point and tragedy had confronted me at every corner. I thought about how I had used that jarring sense of living two lives to protect myself from the pain, how my career had offered a sanctuary from the struggle. That day I played for laughs, and that, at least for a few hours, insulated me from the all-encompassing loss.

There is no doubt that I was totally comforted by the fact that

Mum had died with her beloved son by her side, on his birthday of all days. If she could have dreamt up the perfect death, that would have been it. At home, with her son by her side on his birthday – the very same day that had given new meaning to her life all those years before. Cicely Saunders, the founder of the UK hospice movement, says 'how people die remains in the memory of those who live on'. I knew it in my bones that my lovely mum was at peace and, while my sadness would build exponentially as the reality set in, part of me was at peace with her too.

CHAPTER TEN

Can you make sure, *beta*?

I was encased in a fug of misery.

Every morning that week I woke surprised anew at the lack of tightness across my chest. The leaden, puffy eyes I'd become used to seeing staring back at me in the mirror for months had vanished. Mum passed away on Sunday, 3 November 2019, surrounded by her family. Aside from it being Raj's birthday, my brother had also been scheduled to lead worship at a prayer meeting that day. It felt like serendipity. The service included a puja ceremony, which is a ritual worship where we offer prayers to honour a special person or their memory, or observe an event on a spiritual level, so Mum's passing was immediately recognized and venerated. During the puja a fire is lit, and offerings of flowers and water are made and sweets and food are shared among those attending. That Sunday, the whole family attended temple and my mum's memories were celebrated. Akshay's presence made it feel like there was representation from our side of the family. Though I wasn't there to experience it, I heard that the service was a beautiful thing and I know it helped several members of our family to start to accept what had happened. Everybody wants and needs different things in that moment and for some our religion was a huge support, which is a wonderful thing.

I'm not particularly religious, and Mum was observant rather than dedicated. I used to drop her at the monthly prayer meetings, but I didn't attend them often. I did not wish my mum's relationship with her faith to be sullied by my becoming the focus of community gossip. Religion was always Raj's thing, as he is a devout man. I love all places of worship – synagogues, gurdwaras, churches, mosques and temples – and have a deep respect for those who practise in them. The prayer space on that day was actually the same church hall that I'd learnt to dance in all those years ago, so I will always have a connection to it. But community worship isn't the way that I connect spiritually.

Sincerity is paramount for me; it wouldn't have been honest for me to turn up on that Sunday. Even if I had been in Oldham, I may not have gone. I couldn't now pretend; I had to hold myself accountable to my own truth. I do often think about how much easier things could have been if I could 'go with the flow' a bit more and not be so rigorously sincere. It was a characteristic I'd inherited from Mum – if she had been less tied to her sincerity, perhaps she would have disowned me when I became pregnant, like some of the family had wanted her to do. But she was happy to experience personal discomfort to do what she believed was right. I wasn't as strong as her, or as like her as I wanted to be. She was the strongest of us all.

As the next week came around, the funeral preparations began. I had rehearsals every day in London, but we scheduled FaceTime meetings with the funeral directors to make sure we were all involved. We hadn't been able to find any services which dealt specifically with Hindu funerals in Oldham – there were some Caribbean funeral companies, but nothing that was tailored completely to our culture. Instead we decided to work with funeral directors who had been recommend to us. It turned out the company was owned by one of my old schoolfriends who had joined her family funeral business, so there was at least a connection. The whole process was really difficult because we were all at different points in our grief for our mum. Splitting the decisions four ways among siblings on top of ensuring that my mother's wishes were taken into consideration proved to be as hard as it sounds.

For years, when we'd be sitting in her room, Mum would turn to me and say, **'Shobi, I want to give this to you and can you make sure "so and so" gets this, can you make sure, *beta*?'** At first I'd brush it off, laugh and say she was being silly – this was in the years before we had begun any of the mental health battles. But as she continued to voice these bequests, I told her that she should write them down. I could have done it for her, but it was far better for her to speak to a lawyer and get everything in writing. From around 2010 she began to bring up her own death more often, so I encouraged her to make a proper will. I can remember finding in a book a note that she had written when she went into hospital with bowel cancer in 2014 which simply said, **'When I am gone please let Shobna clear up my house and belongings after me.'** When she got home and began to convalesce I thought it was important to address the issue because of all the potential trouble it could cause. I explained to her that she needed a more formal statement of her will because of my place in the family. Given the family dynamic, it felt that unless things were very clearly – and legally – defined, I might be on unstable ground if I 'self-designated' myself to be the one to uphold her wishes.

In the end she did make a will and wrote a letter of wishes. I think she had wanted it to be me, because I didn't have a husband or a household outside of Akshay to look after. There wasn't a male influence and she knew that I would do exactly as she wanted. Or perhaps, after all this time, she finally recognized the value of this woman next to her. Traditionally the noun '*beta*' would be used to refer exclusively to a son, and daughters would be called '*beti*'. While customs have changed and *beta* is increasingly used to refer to children of both sexes, every time I heard my Mum call me *beta* and registered her apparent lapse in traditional grammar, it felt good. As if finally my gender ceased to matter, and I was as capable as a son. It was of no regard any more that I was her *third* daughter, I was the *beta* that she wanted to put everything right for her when she wasn't here to do it herself.

To smooth any future rifts, I had also said, 'Mum, you need to pick somebody else as well as me to organize everything,' and she had nominated Sushma. In 2017, when she was diagnosed with dementia, Sushma and I became her power of attorney for financial things, while Raj took on that role in medical matters. Taking that step was so hard for all of us. How do you even approach taking responsibility for your parent's decisions?

The spur to address the issue was created by a set of bank charges that had accrued because Mum had been unknowingly going into her overdraft. I had one of the most intense meetings of my life when I went into the bank, Mum in tow, and sat in a room and explained to one of the bank managers what had happened, without explicitly mentioning in front of Mum that she had dementia. I didn't want Mum to feel like she was responsible for it at all. Like when she got stopped by a security guard in Asda because she hadn't paid properly on one of the self-service tills – she hadn't realized it hadn't taken her payment. She hadn't stopped talking for months about how badly she had been treated. She had been spoken to like a petty thief and it caused her real pain that she revisited again and again. I went in to complain to them too, but they really didn't take it on board. I was adamant that Mum wouldn't be treated badly or punished for something that she just couldn't control.

We had discussed the power of attorney question together as a team with Mum. We had to phrase it carefully and we focused very much on her physical condition. 'Mum, if you can't make a decision because you are too ill, who would you like to make those decisions for you?' We still couldn't directly discuss the deterioration of her mind in relation to these affairs. In Mum's lucid moments, she knew it was the right way forward and agreed that the arrangements would be for the best, which helped us all feel more comfortable with the set-up, but it was still really tough.

In Mum's letter of wishes she had been very clear about what she wanted for her last moments on this earth. Mum wasn't piously religious and had always been most fond of attending prayer meetings to preserve her links with the community and her friends, so I wasn't surprised that she said that she didn't want her ashes to be scattered in the Ganges, which would have been the more traditionally religious choice. Her feeling was that as she had been born in the UK and had lived her life here, she was British through and through. **'Like a stick of Blackpool rock, but from Southport,'** she would quip.

Many other Hindus living in Britain want their ashes to be scattered at Varanasi or, as Mum still called it, Benares, the city's former colonial name. Varanasi, on the banks of the Ganges, is the holiest of seven sacred cities in Hinduism. It's written that being cremated along the holy banks of the river will break the cycle of rebirth and reincarnation, so a soul can finally gain salvation, rest in peace and step off that endless cycle of time. Dad's funeral took place on the very banks of the holy River Ganges and his ashes were scattered in the water. But he had died in India and so those religious and cultural expectations took over. Because he had been so young and had died so unexpectedly, no one had really known what his wishes were. Somewhere in the back of my mind regarding my dad, I have always been comforted by the fact that maybe he had died where he wanted to, however suddenly, having returned to his homeland.

For Mum, everything had always centred on staying in her house. She had shored herself up within its walls to weather the storm raging in her mind; this was a place of safety and control and the peace she wanted to find would undoubtedly lie here. She would often talk of how Dad had worked so hard to buy the strip of land and then built the house from scratch. They had chosen every little thing about that house and garden together. Mum wanted to die at home and that was something she expressed before her diagnosis and often in moments of clarity after it too. Mum told us and wrote that she wanted her ashes to be spread in the garden at home and in Southport in the sea, where she was born.

She would say to me, '**What about yours?**' and I'd always say, 'Manchester Ship Canal.' It doesn't sound the most romantic of places, but for me it is another one of the most emblematic landmarks of British history. Whether it was transporting all that cotton and goods from across the world to the northern industrial

towns and cities which powered the 'Great' in Britain, in turn
enabling the forced transportation of millions of African people to
the cotton fields of the southern United States and the Caribbean,
or else carrying the trade of people and goods from the Empire in
India and other colonies, the canal symbolizes our *real* history: the
history of Imperial profit and global domination all built off the
back of desperate exploitation and enslavement. The industrial
town where I was born was central to Britain's growing wealth from
the 1700s due to its position on that trade route, and the canal is the
perfect place for me because I am a small part of that long, hidden,
awful colonial legacy. I'm also anecdotally told that the old canal
runs through the bottom of the old *Coronation Street* set, on Quay
Street. And what can I say? I've got at least a bit of sentimentality for
my years on Mum's favourite soap. She used to laugh at me and say
that Manchester Ship Canal sounded ridiculous, but it still stands.
'Why not?' I would say. 'I want to be in Britain's veins after I'm dead,
just like the ancestors.' She would then nod quietly. What I never
pointed out when she laughed at my not-so-idyllic final place of rest
was that Southport wasn't the most picturesque destination either.
But that was what she wanted.

When it came to what she believed in, it always came back
to dharma and karma. Dharma, the sense of duty and the right
way of living, and karma, the spiritual connection between cause
and effect. That belief was implicit in her favourite phrase, **'What
have I done to deserve this?'** Whether it be Dad's death or her
health problems, or having a daughter who turned out like me,
she would always talk about her bad karma from a past life. **'What
must have happened for me to deserve this life?'** Hindu religion
teaches that when we die, our soul passes into another body, but
I'm not sure if Mum was completely sold on that, karma or no
karma. What she did definitely believe was that when she died she

would meet Dad again. She would say she didn't know where he was or how they would meet, but she trusted to her core that they would be together again. She had waited so patiently for 35 years to be reunited with him.

The question was how we could fit her wishes in with the traditions of our faith and the ways each of us wanted to honour her too. It's not an easy thing to bring everyone together when resentments and feelings of hurt are so close to the surface, but I was determined that we would present the family in the way that Mum would have wanted. People grieve differently and express loss in unpredictable ways, so you have to let things go, and we managed somehow to do that for her. It was like she was there with us, guiding us away from the bubbling animosities and into the shallows of ceasefire.

Hema rallied everyone from India, and worldwide. Raj contacted the local and wider community of Mum's and Dad's friends in the UK, and we spoke with her friends from all of her charitable groups. Mum dying brought us all together to perform, like we had so many times in our childhood, for that one final show. I've always been the one to write among my siblings, so I volunteered to put together the eulogy and take that off everybody's shoulders. It felt like I was in effect still 'working away', because writing is something you can do anywhere.

It felt like a natural way for me to contribute and I was pleased that everyone else could go ahead and focus on other things. It's incredibly daunting to write something which is supposed to encapsulate and honour a person's life, especially when you are one of many who love them so much. I wanted to do her justice and make sure it was impartial, so I asked everyone, my immediate siblings first and the wider family and friends from all generations, to contribute their memories and stories. Even

though I was writing the eulogy, I wanted to try and erase myself
from it. I felt safer hiding myself and my own recollections of her
and instead painted her picture through the stories of others. I
didn't want anyone to think that I had tried to take over, or that I'd
wanted to steal the attention from Mum.

The process made me reflect on what these memories meant.
The little slips of paper, WhatsApp messages and emails sent from
the furthest seas, which all of our closest friends and family had
scrawled or typed to share their personal vignettes of my mum.
All the memories she had shared with me, those windows into
who she was: Mum and Dad coming to England, her recollections
of her childhood, Blighty in the war-torn 1940s and then in the
Swinging Sixties. All her journeys across the world. Everything
she had shared with us.

What did they really mean? When someone dies, I wondered,
are the memories about the person we try so hard to cling on
to or are they actually more about the person remembering?
The chasm between life and death seems so narrow, especially
when your strongest link to the world, the woman who gave
you life itself, falls away. I sometimes felt like I was living in a
twilight – it became hard to hold on to my own belief systems,
and to register what were my memories and what I had created
of her that I found in me or from the stories I had collected from
everyone else. I relied on one of my friends, Charles, to help me
decipher my thoughts. He knew Mum and me, and I had called
him on numerous other occasions when I had public speaking
engagements. He encouraged me just to 'write everything down',
instead of it swirling around in my head.

On the Friday after she died, I boarded the train from London
back home in a haze. I spent the journey working on the logistics

of the funeral and plotted it all minute by minute. The pandit would start by leading us in prayer, give his thoughts and then recite the Gayatri Mantra, a Sanskrit prayer which through regular chanting is thought to have the power to calm the mind while removing toxins from the body. It also happened to be Mum's go-to mantra. Then there would be a minute's silence, which would complete the first ten minutes. Hema and her girls would follow with a song, three minutes, the eulogy had to be done within twenty minutes after that, to give enough time for Akshay's reading, two minutes, Raj's song for Mum, five minutes, one of Hema's daughters' poem, three minutes, and an ensemble song that we would all sing together for Mum at the end.

There had been a bit of upset towards the end of the planning, as I wasn't sure that everything would fit into the time slot allocated for the service so I had asked everyone to be flexible around their contribution. I wasn't saying that my role was more important, but instead that Mum should be centre stage. Her eulogy would keep the spotlight fixed on her. By this point, my other cousins from abroad had arrived and the whole family insisted on hearing what I had written before I read it on the day. My contribution had to be vetted. I'm not sure if it was because they didn't trust me, the family's 'anomaly', or perhaps they just wanted to make sure I had got all of it in. Either way, I openly shared it, even though no one else contributing did the same. I felt the pinprick of distrust, but kept focused on the fact that it was all for Mum, nothing else mattered.

The day itself was a still, clear day of sunshine. It was unusually seasonable for Oldham in November. Mum always used to say if you had the last spoon of food from the dish or you scraped the pan out and ate every last morsel, '**it would rain on your wedding day**'.

I couldn't get this memory of her voice out of my head. I could feel our silent laughter in that warm sunshine, us both wordlessly shaking. Mum had so often had the last spoon and scraped a bowl or pan clean...yet miraculously it didn't rain on her wedding day nor indeed did it on this day, the day of her funeral.

Before the cremation there was a ceremony at home, so Mum was brought back to her house early that morning. One of my cousins had said our ways were slightly antiquated for modern Indians. Customs there have moved on since we moved to this country, or maybe within our small community in the north of England, we keep a tighter hold on the standards we once knew. There had been little discussion about it – Mum would have an open coffin, as is customary, and would need to be dressed to make her final presentation to the world.

I hadn't seen Mum since I had said my final goodbye. The others had all been there when she died, but for me this was the first time I had seen her with my own eyes afterwards. There was no fear on seeing her dead. I know it's a cliché but she looked so peaceful, as if she were asleep.

In the same way I had done so many times in life, I dressed Mum, but this time I knew it would be the last time I would do so. For years I'd been picking out things for her to wear because she'd forgotten what she owned. The pandit wanted her to wear her wedding sari, as is tradition, but as a family we made the decision that, while it would be right to put something from Dad and their wedding into her coffin, as her memories from that day and of him had faded so completely by the end it would be better to dress her in something she had really loved right up until she left this world. Whenever Mum had gone 'out out' she had always worn an exquisite sari. Always. If she was just going out, it would be a salwar kameez, but if it was anything remotely special, it would be a sari.

This was to be her final outing in this world, so we decided to dress her in the last thing I had put out for her before she stopped going out, her latest sari. I had always helped my mum with her pleats, which are the most complicated part of a sari. You start by pre-folding evenly from the length of the sari and tuck this into the waist, with the final length wrapped around your body covering your midriff, then draped in more folds elegantly across one shoulder. Mum had always helped me with my pleating too, right back to when I was dancing in 'half saris'. It's a tricky thing to get right. To get even and neat pleats with a traditional sari, which is a whole nine yards of material, takes experience, and it's always useful to have someone there to help you fold it into place.

The process of dressing my mother was where we found closeness as a mother and daughter; the preparation of an outfit and helping one another into the 'out out' outfits always felt very tender, full of love and tradition. It had also been a part of our falling out at that wedding in India, all those years before. I will never forget her refusing to help with my sari because she was so cross with me. It was something that had always been special between us, so it cut deeply. Now though, all thoughts of that were gone from my head and my only desire was to get it just right for her as I had always done. The funeral directors were concerned I would be 'too upset' to see it through, but I felt calm and grateful to be able to do this for her.

After her sari was perfect, I moved on to her make-up, which also felt natural because I'd been helping her apply her face and style her hair for such a long period of our lives. That was also always something I'd done within our family – I had done both of my sisters' make-up for their weddings. It was another one of those set roles we all have and hardly think about until you realize it is the final time. I'd bought Mum a new red lipstick and some nail polish, and my sisters carefully painted her nails one by one. It was a sparkly glitter polish over a deep red base, her absolute favourite. It was a difficult process, but it felt like a fitting way for us to care for our mother, helping to prepare her for what was next – who else would have done but her girls?

She'd let me be there for her for so long and she had known I was going to look after her right up to the end, and that made me feel a deep sense of contentment. It was my duty for this last time and when I'd finished, she looked so beautiful and calm. Gone was the look of the disease or worry, she was just ready for the next stage of her journey. After our life of dramas, the trauma had evaporated from her mind and face.

Mum in death,
Mum in life,
Mum in health,
Mum in ill health,
Mum as a girl,
Mum as a friend,
Mum as a wife,
Mum as a daughter,
Mum as a sister,
Mum as a woman,
Mum as a nani,
Mum as an aunty,
Mum with dementia,
Mum as Mum,
They were all there,
Each avatar,
All were Mum.

Although it was distressing knowing that she was no longer there, I felt completely at ease in her presence. I knew that we had given her everything that she'd hoped for in death. I didn't feel that there was anything missing for her.

But I did miss her.

I missed her saying **'cup of tea?'** And her smiling at me saying, **'please?'**

I missed my memories of her shouting, from another room, to fill the water up to the top hole of the teapot. Or calling me a donkey, pig or owl.

Or being a *namoona* for being ungroomed.

Yet most of the memories are good memories. I didn't mind the bad ones any more.

The family and close friends gathered for the ceremony in the living room that was once her bedroom and we all walked around her open coffin, putting in things that she would need in the next life as the pandit led the prayers. There were practicalities like water and food such as sweetmeats, as well as beautiful flowers, incense, and also memories of this life including her wedding shawl as a nod to tradition. I used to keep a crystal in Mum's house, one that my friend had given me for protection. I used to wash it, bless it every full moon cycle, and hide it in her kitchen to keep her safe. When it came to my turn, I put that crystal in as my final bid to protect her.

Then we heard the hearse pull up and she was conveyed into the car as her neighbours next to and across from came out to say goodbye. It was an incredible thing to see and experience, that outpouring of love all around the home she had so loved for so much of her life. We had two flower arrangements, one reading 'Asha' and another spelling out 'OM', the sacred sound of the universe, the eternal spiritual symbol of creation, preservation and liberation.

Days before, there had been heated conversations about
whether we should ask for flowers or donations, and the latter
was decided upon because Mum had always been so keenly
philanthropic. The next issue had been about where the
donations would go to.

Our mother had been very proud and hadn't wanted anyone
to find out about her dementia, it had remained taboo and kept
behind closed doors for her right until the end. Sushma wanted
to protect Mum's view and felt that we shouldn't bequeath to
Alzheimer's Research UK. Yet we felt it important to be honest.
I couldn't in good faith write her eulogy without saying she had
dementia, however difficult it was. Sushma conceded and we
agreed that such a donation would be a fitting acknowledgement
of the need to start breaking down any 'shame' while also helping
other families in similar situations. The donations were eventually
shared between Alzheimer's Research UK and Dr Kershaw's
Hospice. By saying it out loud, in front of friends and family, we
would be releasing Mum and the rest of us from all the secrecy
and inhibitions within the community.

On that day, we presented a united front. It would be
nearly the last time some of us would be together in the same
room. It was as if the force of our mum bound us on that day. She
was again the lynchpin with the power to overcome everything.
Through shame, illegitimacy, death, heartbreak and family
breakdown, her force still pulled us together, even when family
history threatened to drive us apart. It was extraordinary. I
imagine what she would have felt had she seen us all there, this
vibrant, cultural, White, Black and Brown family, some partners
and all her children, all of her grandchildren, standing tall in her
honour, the woman who had been the centre of all our worlds.
Carrying Mum's small coffin into the crematorium were two

cousin brothers; Soren, my brother-in-law; Rohan, my nephew;
Akshay, my son; Raj and his son, Roshan. All of us were groomed
and polished, dressed in the traditional white of mourning, with
our earrings gleaming and our hair brushed just so. Of course,
she wouldn't have *said* anything, but just knowing that she wasn't
berating you for letting the family down was enough to know she
was proud. We were all 'well turned out'.

The service was absolutely heaving, literally bursting at the seams,
with people from every generation from all over the world, all over
the country, crushed into the room. Many of them stood through
the whole hour because there wasn't enough seating. That is how
many people she had touched. The cards we'd printed for the
service, with a beautiful picture of her on the front and back and
her favourite prayer written underneath, fluttered in the hands of
our global community. Seeing her face repeated across the crowd
gave me the strength to walk up to the raised stage and address the
mourners.

Throughout the ceremony I had my hand on each person's
back as each of them stood and spoke and sang or cried. I felt
myself click into performance mode. 'Leave your shit and your
chewing gum at the door,' as one teacher used to say, advice
that has always stayed with me. There should be no ego in
performance. It's my harbour in every storm and the rush of
adrenalin switched every synapse on and up to the max. The
performance was never mine, it was Asha's. Everything passed in a
blur, my heart racing as I tried to engage in the shape of the words.
It felt like time had suddenly started to play again and we were in
fast-forward, the total opposite of the 'paused' long, languorous
days I had spent with Mum. And, before I could exhale, we
were at the final song. As one, we harmonized The Beatles' 'All

My Loving', changing the 'my' to 'our'. It was triumphant and transcendent – this ivory-clad choir mourning but rejoicing in our matriarch, who would never leave our side.

In Hindu culture, the final rites are always performed by the eldest son, and in the same way as he had been expected to take those heavy steps on the banks of the Ganges for his father at just 14 years of age, it was Raj's role to make the final action to press the button which would commit Mum's body into the flames. I felt so strongly that it shouldn't be all his responsibility, that this patriarchal attitude which seeps through so much of our society and organized religion was palpably wrong. When it came to it, I remember leaving my son, despite his distress at the time, and feeling like something was invisibly pulling me like a magnet to my brother. As I stood beside him, I slipped my hand under his and we did it together. No matter how he might have felt about me then, no matter what his thoughts in the past or what he feels today, no matter that we will never speak again, at that juncture I felt so strongly that I needed to be there for him. It reminds me of the little girl at temple who used to ask all the questions and demand to know why on earth Sita would walk though fire to prove herself. These rigid rubrics leave families torn, separated from each other when they need each other most. At the end, I wanted to share the burden with my brother even though it broke the rules, and the pandit didn't mind.

And then it was over. Mum's coffin went into the flames of the oven. There was an acute feeling of hopelessness.

It shook us all to the core.

And then you step outside and feel the sun warm your skin and you realize with trepidation that it's your job to speak to people who have come to comfort you and find comfort for themselves, when you have no words left to give anyone. The moments you have just experienced will take you weeks, months, years to reconcile into a memory. It slowly dawns on you that it is over.

There were so many faces from the past and present. Old and new. The greatest surprise had been the arrival of my mum's younger brother, the one she had been estranged from. We spoke for a short while and I thanked him for coming. It was the respect that she deserved. Then there was a desperate desire to separate myself from everything, an instinctive need to draw unbreathed air deep down into my lungs.

After the cremation we moved to a hall in Ashton-under-Lyne that was attached to a temple; there is an arbitrary rule that you can't eat and congregate inside temple after a cremation as it is said you would be covered in the ashes of the dead. Raj and Sushma had hired a Gujarati caterer, and they had carefully planned it so there would be some of Mum's favourite dishes that Jayshiri had often made for her. One she had always savoured was dhokla, a steamed cake made from the paste of ground chickpea and rice flour, fermented overnight in warm water and sour yoghurt, topped with coriander and tempered with fried green chilli, mustard seeds and a curry leaf tarka. We realized that we would need a car for ferrying some last-minute bits, so I took the opportunity to step out of the day and set off with my friend Aulton to fetch it.

Aulton was another one of my friends who had become Mum's, as he had helped her around her house with shopping, and moving her boxes and bags of papers from room to room, when I was away. In turn, he credited my mum with bringing him out of a deep depression by sending him a note to check on him one day because she hadn't seen him for a period of time. She'd signed the note: **'Best wishes, always Asha Gulati (Shobi's mum)'**. She had meant a lot to him and I needed him to help us again that day.

Often, when Aulton came to do odd jobs, I'd direct him to what needed fixing as soon as he came through the door. Mum would then shout from the living room, **'Shobi, can't he have a cup of tea first? And while you're at it, I'll have one too, and biscuits please, make sure you put them nicely on a plate.'**

That window of fetching my car diluted the intensity of emotion, and when I arrived at the hall I felt more able to be present. Absolutely everybody wanted to tell me a story about my mum. Many of them mentioned her quick wit and a fondness for jokes, like this joke my cousin sister Vandita had messaged me from her home in America. The gag is about the medical encounters Vandita and her husband had experienced as interns in a hospital in Mumbai. It had been one of mum's favourites – so much so I had added it to the eulogy. A *bhaiya* (an affectionate term meaning brother) comes to A&E. He says to Vandita, *'Chuha kaata'* (a rat bit me), so she immediately asks *'Kahan?'* (Where?) To which the brother replies *'Dhobitallow mein.'* For those unfamiliar with Indian cities, Dhobitallow is a place in Mumbai, not a body part.

It wasn't the joke itself that Vandita remembered so fondly, but more how her Aunty Asha would always burst out laughing before the punchline. Every time she saw her, Mum would ask her to repeat the *'chuha* joke', and before her niece even started Mum would be shaking and snorting uncontrollably with laughter. Vandita finished her story by telling me that the last time she had seen my mum, two years before she died, Mum's memory was clouded and Vandita wasn't sure if Mum remembered her. They had chatted like old friends but my cousin sister wasn't sure if she could place her or knew her name. 'But then with a twinkle in her eye,' Vandita explained, 'she asked, **"Can you tell me the chuha joke?"** At that point, I knew I must occupy a tiny spot somewhere deep in her heart and mind. Aunty Asha, the *chuha* joke is for you. When life's problems get to me, I remember how you laughed at the smallest thing in the hardest of times.'

Other memories of Mum poured in. My friend Shaila remembered meeting Mum at the house and her cooking a South Indian dish of uppama (made of semolina and nuts) as a thoughtful nod to Shaila's heritage. She told me, 'What I recall is a woman with a soft voice but resolute heart – an iron fist in a velvet glove. I admire that quality. Your mother was class: elegant, informed, intelligent and independent. That is how I will remember her.'

Mum had also served on the adoption panel for Oldham Council, was a governor at a local primary school, taught English as a foreign language and put on night-school cookery lessons for adult education. For these, she'd plan her lessons in fine detail, teaching ingredient quantities and exacting methods. Colin Green, one her students, fondly recalled making samosas with her. Daunted by all the steps, he said, 'This must take you ages at home to prepare.' To which Mum glibly responded, **'No Colin, ready-made. I buy them, I fry them.'**

Mum had always been a tireless fundraiser and loved getting dressed up for balls or dinners with Dad. After he passed, I later had the opportunity to take her to celebrity bashes, and I absolutely cherished her being my plus one. Her Inner Wheel functions or my charity dinners would always occupy a space on the calendar that hung in her room, and we would point to the dates to keep her going and give her something to look forward to. As we were reminiscing, another friend, David, recalled meeting Mum at one of our many fancy fundraising dos. He reminded me of one evening when Mum had found herself sitting next to Manchester's very own 'controversial commentator', Terry

Christian. Terry speaks very quickly and has a strong Manchester accent, so I'd been concerned initially about how they would get on, but from across the table their conversation had seemed animated. When David enquired what they were talking about Mum didn't beat about the bush: **'I have no idea what he's saying, I just smile and nod.'** Others spoke of their recollections of just 'how cool' our family was, specifically Mum and Dad, who in comparison to their more rigid parents were much more relaxed. Countless people told me how much they would look forward to Aunty Asha's parties and being part of the more laid back atmosphere in our household.

As the groaning platters were emptied and the line of well-wishers diminished, it was time to pack up and load the scant leftovers into my car. We all were well trained: **'Nothing must go to waste'**. There were no hitches, nothing to regret. No one fell out on that day, no cross words were spoken. We were the family she had always hoped we would be, at our very best.

A few days later we held an intimate religious ceremony with the pandit, in the family home, to absolve Mum of all her sins, and each of us said everything that we needed to say to bid her a final goodbye. The rationale behind this final parting is that these words are to set the soul free. As it was a religious rite my brother led the ceremony, but I was right by his side, my hand underneath his, doing the necessary rituals as the pandit led the service.

A week later we took Mum's ashes to where she was born at the Christiana Hartley Maternity Hospital in Southport. These days it's a GP surgery, but we looked up pictures on the internet of what it would have looked like during the war when Mum was born there, and imagined what it must have been like for her parents as they cradled their little first-born with a full head of hair, **'not bald**

like the other babies', in that quaint seaside town. Afterwards, we went to the edge of the pier and scattered her ashes into the sea, as she had requested. Hema had her eldest daughter with her, I had Akshay with me and Raj and Sushma had their whole families with them.

In true Gulati fashion, after some moments of silence and reflection and photographs, our thoughts went to food – it's in our cultural make-up – and we went for fish and chips before we drove home and spread the remainder of her ashes in her garden. It also happened to be the day before Mum and Dad's Golden Wedding Anniversary, joining up unexpectedly (as it was not planned this way), her cycle of memories.

I still keep this spot in the garden tidy and presentable, as though I am still caring for her, while also trying to restore order in my mind from the grief of her passing. Every month I take flowers and say my words to her in private homage, still by her side because she is there. I choose brightly coloured blooms, which she was always so fond of, constantly finding colour in the greyness in her life. Perhaps this house will be kept in the family for ever. No other family has ever lived in it. For now, it's the place where I go to feel at ease and I often stay over in my bed there, even though there is no one to look after or cajole into getting up in the morning. There are no curtains to open or secret piles of ironing to do. No food to cook. No TV to watch. The purpose and duty I once had has departed, never to return. But I still feel the pull to be there in case I am needed.

I was ready to let her go. I don't know where she is now, but I like to think that the woman who was always right in life was correct in her unshakable belief that in death she would find my father. I think of them together, this time never to be parted, as I sit in the house they built, looking through the photographs of all the memories they had together and the life they worked hard to create for us. I think that I have started to put back together the lost mind of my mother, and that I will keep coming back here and combing over it all until I do. It is my last rite for her, without ceremony, but as a dedication to her being the person who prevented my own life from falling apart.

Mum was indeed the personification of the meaning of her name: hope. She gave me that 'brimful of Asha'.

Remember me?

It has been three months since I last took a deep, full breath;
twelve weeks since I've been able to walk up the stairs instead of
scrabbling up them using my arms and hands; a quarter of a year
since I first woke in the night, bed drenched with sweat, with a
fever raging and the certainty that I'd been infected with the virus
that had been burning, unchecked, through our cities, exploiting
every weakness in our society. Poor people? Old people? Disabled
people? People with Black and Brown heritage? Covid-19 and
a government which has for so long failed to protect our most
vulnerable have no qualms.

I find myself locked into an eerie state of isolation, while
simultaneously feeling ever more connected to my mother, both
when she first suffered after being widowed and then when her

body and mind failed her at the end of her life. I have become even more acutely sensitive to that part of her. The struggle against this virus which retreats only to regroup has felt relentless; the hospital visits and virtual GP consultations never seem to lead to a resolution.

When I first saw the doctor she looked me up and down before telling me that she couldn't test me as testing was not the policy the NHS were following (intimating but not confirming that the government were leading with 'herd immunity'). Despite the risks to herself – though masked and aproned, she couldn't practise social distancing while listening to my chest – she also informed me that I had a secondary bacterial infection of pneumonia and prescribed a course of strong antibiotics.

It is only now I realize that without her on the frontline of the NHS, this dutiful, diligent duty doctor of Nigerian parentage, I may not have survived. I am forever grateful for her brilliant insight on that fateful day in early March. Months later came the eventual diagnosis from an antibody test. I was alone, but many of my 'minority' were also struck down. Everywhere I looked, friends and family were being unequally felled by this ruthless disease.

When the streets of people opened their front doors to clap for the NHS, I could hear my mother's voice, wryly saying, **'Are they clapping for us now?'** She would marvel at the irony of how hard her husband had worked in the NHS and how hard her son was working now without any public acclaim. My father and brother channelled an incredible work ethic and level of skill to work in our health industry despite all the prejudice, pay gaps and glass ceilings. But now, in fighting our current pandemic, the abilities clearly needed are so often provided by people who are cast to the fringes of popular attention and privilege. The so-called 'low-skilled' are at the frontline in this national emergency too. My mum's dry comments would note that underpinning this clapping was the nation's ignorance of the very real contributions our families has made over the last century, as well as those who came on the *Empire Windrush* to aid the building of our national treasure, the NHS. And now, sadly, it is us again, and this time dying in disproportionate numbers from Covid-19 on that frontline.

Do you think you know me?

Everyone presumes they know my upbringing because of the colour of my skin. People who know nothing of my actual background, my mother, her parents, the story of Empire and my son don't ask, they just believe their own assumptions. I remember showing an ITV exec a picture of my grandmother as I asked about the lack of Black and Brown actors in period drama. My grandmother lived in wartime Britain, and dressed accordingly – in a tweed skirt and jacket and with a bindi on her forehead. The TV exec was palpably shocked. People presume to know my heritage, locked into their stereotype of what a 'BAME' person is. I've always hated labels that mean absolutely nothing to the people they describe. I remember when I first read that I was 'BAME' – a political abbreviation for people from Black, Asian and Minority Ethnic backgrounds – I thought you pronounced it like 'game' but with a 'b'. To the people who come up with these acronyms, perhaps it is a game. When I found out it was meant to encompass the experiences of any non-white person, as if anyone with high melanin was this homogenous group, it made me want to scream at the newspaper. It's just another example of how people think they know your story based on your skin tone.

Colour prejudice is very much a part of my and Akshay's lived experience. In 2001, when Oldham had a period of significant racially-motivated violence, my own home was daubed with 'white rules' across the front of the house. It was hard to take on board. Mum's reaction was, **'Just clean it off, *beta*, they don't know what they're saying.'** Her rather sanguine approach – to **'wash it away'** – was how she first responded when, in 1964, she appeared as a model in the local paper. The rather suspect headline, 'When sari wife taps on fashion's door', was accompanied by commentary along the lines that, although nobody will admit an actual colour bar, it's only a few organizations that will 'engage any dark-skinned beauties'.

Years later, I'm conscious of how much more upset my mum was in response to being 'othered', when Akshay was first stopped and searched, and when he had 'Oi, ISIS' shouted at him in the street. She constantly worried about how his cultural heritage was viewed by certain corners of society and some of those in authority, and how this combination could end up getting him killed. He was on her mind more than anybody else in the months before she died. I imagine her to have completely understood why Black lives matter.

Mum died just before we headed into winter. I sleepwalked through Christmas; the start of spring was supposed to herald a new chapter. In the past, whenever I was due to start a new tour, and whenever I travelled, Mum would ask me to call her when I arrived. As I've already said, even if I was just leaving hers to go back down the road to my house, she'd say the same: **'Call me when you get home, Shobi.'** I'd always laugh and say, 'Mum, I'm just going around the corner,' but still, I always did it. She'd invariably pick up and say, **'OK, fine. I'm glad you're there,'** then hang up before you could even reply, quickly getting back to her TV so she wouldn't miss any of the programme she was following. She just always wanted to know I was safe. Wherever I was in the world, I made sure I checked in with her as soon as I got to my hotel, so she always knew where I was. She would note down the landline – she was not keen on mobile phones, and once said, 'I don't want one of those, I don't want any of you keeping tabs on me.' When I went down to London to start back at work, there was no one to call. When the tour started, and I made it to Sheffield or Edinburgh, there was no one to phone when I arrived. No one to send a postcard to. That person who always wanted to know I was safe has gone. I *was* safe, but no one knew I was.

And then I got very sick indeed. Even in the moments when I was most ravaged by this illness, which crept into my life and home as an unexpected visitor and has decided to keep me hostage with no promise of a ransom, I could hear my mother saying, 'Well, I don't really like people and I don't go outside anyway, it's too cold. You need to keep your distance and stay warm.'

I also felt a strange sense of role reversal as all my senses began to fade, just as hers had. Sometimes I would make her something to eat and she'd take a tiny taste and say, '*Beta*, I forgot to put salt in, can you bring some?' Even then she still believed that it was her mistake, as she had thought she'd cooked the meal. I had always been so disappointed that she didn't like what I'd worked so hard to make her, especially when I knew that I'd already added plenty of love and seasoning. But now that I've experienced that total sensory loss, I can understand exactly why she rejected what I'd made her – she may have had no taste at all on occasions due to respiratory illness or medication. How I wish I could have known this back then. But that's perspective.

And, of course, Mum in my mind tells me it is my fault I caught the virus. 'Shobi, you should have washed your hands properly with soap in the first place.' I tell her it's not for a want of hand washing. What she never realized was how much she had rubbed off on me. Akshay has always complained about being harangued by me to 'take your dirty outside clothes off before you sit on the sofa, you have to change into house clothes first' the moment he arrives at mine. And this was BC, before Covid-19!

Over these months of reflection, I have realized that this woman who for so many years I failed to please has shaped every edge and contour of the woman I am today. While I certainly have my own eccentricities, underneath the veil of independence I'm very much like her, just 26 years younger – even down to my 'Rear of the Year 2012' behind (as a cheeky aside, no pun intended, but I got it from my mama). In addition to our mutual obsession with fairness and sincerity, I've also realized I am not the most demonstrative person when it comes to emotion. Recently Akshay told me he loved me and I found myself struggling to say it back. It took me a long while to get there. It's not for the lack of love but because of the coding installed in me. He always asks me if I want to hug, as though he has to ask permission. He never gives up, and we do hug. And now all I do in lockdown is long for one, and for my mother to hold my 'clean' hands through this painful passage too. When we become parents, we make that unsaid promise to ourselves to be 'better than' our parents, but without proper self-examination we invariably find ourselves in exactly in the same place as them.

I've tried really hard not to bring some of the hurt of the past with me. Yes, I was a single mum because things had not worked out with Akshay's dad and that created an extremely challenging set of personal circumstances. Akshay and I have had some tumultuous times over the years and I suppose those will continue as we grow together as mum and son.

Right at the outset, I remember the registrar tutting as I wrestled with whether to put Akshay's father on the birth certificate. But I did, and I have always felt that it's important to recognize that Akshay has a dad and shares a family heritage with him, even if he was absent in his early life. I would have liked to have enjoyed the highs and lows of parenting with his dad but that just wasn't our path, and anyway my mum became really good at sharing our celebrations. I took my personal hurt out of the father–son equation. It wasn't the easiest thing to do and I wasn't always good at that. I wanted to make sure that, even though he was my ex, he would never be erased from Akshay's life, and as the years have passed, father and son have spent time together. Akshay has always been welcome and a part of his dad's family. Equally, Akshay has always been taken into the hearts of all my siblings, their families and their children. Loving him was never in question for them, despite what some of them may think of me. Indeed I've continued to encourage those close relationships. So you see, I do try to work things out as I go along – just as my mum showed her duty towards me, it was my duty as Akshay's mum.

Not only have I inherited and passed on Mum's fierce duty to her family, but also her aversion to any prejudice. While our childhoods were – quite literally – worlds apart, her route to feminism, the way she challenged herself to confront the limitations of her experience, took her on a journey that reflected my own, and we managed to find commonality in this space we had both fostered within ourselves. It also feels like I have started to inhabit her role – in lockdown, Sushma has called to say, 'I used to ring Mum for recipes and now I ring you.' My physicality is similar to my mum's too, I'm told that I am looking more and more like her, and share her almost unnatural ability to look fresh-faced and healthy even in the depths of debilitating health crises. 'How do you look so young and glowing when you've got Covid-19?' Sushma asks over FaceTime. 'You look so much like Mum always did, it's weird.' I think perhaps it's good lighting from the window, or that we both just really miss her.

Of course, there are also elements of the cultural conditioning which Mum carried throughout her life that I feel I must let go of now. A lot of the shame and trauma she held so tightly have no place in my life or this world I find myself living in. The belief that she deserved the tragedies that befell her isn't part of my worldview. I want to reconcile my own mistakes and missteps, especially as I know that a lack of self-forgiveness leads me to a place where I am not able to protect myself. In that void, as George Eliot says, 'cruelty...only requires opportunity', which takes me into self-harm, and in some of my previous relationships this has been characterized by a vicious cycle of abuse, gaslighting and ghosting. Yet I do sometimes catch myself still chiming in with Mum and Nazar, so every time my son gets a compliment I fight off this 'evil eye', saying, 'Oh yes, thank you, he's lovely, but he's a right pain in the neck.' I have kept some of the idiosyncrasies but not the shame/*sharam*, the more embedded patriarchal and societal conditioning rendered on our family. I have a piece of pop art by the Canadian artist Maria Qamar (@Hatecopy), which depicts an image of an Indian woman with a speech bubble saying 'Has anyone seen my sharam?' I enjoy that work of art, and I am pleased to report that my *sharam* is lost, for ever.

The years I cared for Mum will shape my life and perhaps change the course of it. The time we spent together will make me live a different way when there's living to be done outside my four walls. I have decided I'll be more fearless: I'll face the consequences of writing this book and the admissions I've made here and what that will mean for my reputation and position in my community. Or in my family. Because what she and I went through – away from the public eye, in the private inner sanctum of her home – has forced me to understand why we need to accept our own story; to understand that our own perspective and voice are valuable.

We went on a journey together, she and I, finding our own paths in life. You never think about your parents as still-evolving, because as a child you need to rely on them to remain exactly the same as the cornerstones of your existence. Having your own children exposes the faults in that logic, but the past 25 years with my mum, watching how she changed and discovered and lost parts of herself, revealed to us that your worth and value will never be found in other people's eyes. It can only be found in yourself. And you have to learn to trust that. My mum lived her life like that.

Shortly after she passed away, my brother revealed his true feelings to me. I had just come off stage from a performance and was getting ready to go to my digs. I had put him on loudspeaker in my dressing room and I couldn't really take in what he was saying. He said that there was no forgiveness for what I was, what I had done, who I had become or where I was going. Though I knew his words were steeped in his grief, my suspicion that he had been keeping his true feelings about me locked away out of respect for Mum had been correct. I am determined this family rupture will not shake my self-acceptance. Though I do understand that, at some point in life, I will have to admit that all of us siblings have been on our own individual journeys, and that I will one day want to reconcile my feelings of hurt to keep that promise I made to my mum as she was dying – for us to be the family once again, the one she remarkably kept together along the way, despite everything that had happened to fracture our lives.

Caring for Mum, dealing with our grief and sharing the responsibility of Mum's affairs have brought me and my sister, Sushma, to a deeper mutual understanding. And so with her, I can now be freed from how my family remembers me. I don't want to 'walk through fire' to absolve myself of any sin, imagined or real. I can see myself as the small girl asking about Ram, and questioning Sita in the story Ramayana, but now I am grown and I have my own answers.

Mum's death has brought the conviction that I don't want to seek that validation from anyone any more. Five decades of seeking validation from the outside has led only to pain and emotional turmoil. Now I see my truth. I'm not ashamed of what I have done. If you label it as misbehaviour, that is something to do with you and your perception. As the educator Dennis Kimbro says, 'Our perception is shaped by our previous experiences.' So really, it's nothing to do with me, it's **'water off a duck's back'** – one of my mum's favourite English idioms, when anyone tried to harm her.

Just as Mum inhabited different parts of her whole person as she lost her mind, I too want to put parts of myself to rest at last and start looking back without shame in order to look further out. If that means I will be estranged from those with whom I share blood, or friends that I once loved, so be it.

From those years of caring for Mum, my biggest lesson has been that patience is the key to everything. Previously, I had been the most impatient person, even with myself. Though this has fuelled my ambition, it has also driven me damagingly off course. It serves no purpose to be frustrated with what you can't control. Yes, there is only one destination, and the path you take to that end is much more important and significant than the inevitable end itself.

The journey with Mum was remarkable as we dipped into pools of memory afresh and tasted things which transported us to forgotten conversations and moments. I followed her as she adventured in her past, as if the more she lost the greater clarity was given to what remained. I was a passenger strapped alongside her as we drove out together into her mind, where we learnt to forget the present and to disregard the future. This was our time, like those times we had shared in her car when I was a young girl, the place where we could safely cross boundaries in the topics we discussed.

No one wants to be there at the conclusion of a terminal illness. Stepping onboard and giving in to the inexorable, uncontrollable journey of taking care of Mum at the end has been one of the most defining experiences of my life.

In many 'non-western' cultures, worth is put on age because it is seen as the way to accumulate knowledge and wisdom, both of which afford you respect. But here in the west some reject the old. Their status in our society is dust. And should they have the misfortune to suffer from dementia, that standing is even further depleted.

What did they ever know?

Why listen to someone who has forgotten how to do the simple tasks of everyday life?

What value can they hold now?

What is their use?

What can they contribute to us?

What is their function?

The taboos and anxiety around dementia exist because our elderly also fear losing the last sliver of social value they are clinging on to. In many ways, I hope that the Covid-19 outbreak highlights this cultural indignity and inequity. I hope that we will stay outraged about the way our mothers and fathers have been allowed to die. Make no mistake, the disregard for our vulnerable is political.

Older people are not expendable, they should not be treated as a burden, though of course caring *is* a job. But our society isn't built for us to care for our elderly parents. We are just about coming around to finding space for childcare in certain professions, but elderly care hasn't been afforded the same spotlight among professionals in the workplace or with the politicians who make the rules. I can remember going into jobs and telling prospective employers that I cared for my mum. I'd ask if it were possible to find me a parking space in case I had to travel at short notice, or to have flexible days during rehearsals and have some early weekends off. Some theatres rehearsals can start at 11am – if you have children to get to school, that's great, but if that means a late finish, you're not going to be able to be there for an elderly parent in another part of the country without difficulty. But trying to find these solutions constantly makes you feel like an inconvenience – I can only imagine how the elderly person you're caring for might feel.

As I write in the middle of this crisis, we can see we have failed our elderly. It's the difference between caring and not caring, and the problem for carers is that they're currently doing their job in a society where the majority of people and those with power don't really care. The protective ring around our care homes the government said they were implementing didn't really protect anyone after all.

I believe that Mum's with me and I carry her into all I do. I know I'm grieving but, as strange as it might sound, she feels less lost to me now than when she had dementia. I know that she was physically present during those years, but on many of those days she was so far from herself and from me, I couldn't reach her in the way that I can now. Part of me feels that in her peace, St Anthony has lifted the layers of her confusion, reunited her with the lost parts of herself she asked him to find for her and brought her back to me.

No longer do I have to worry about whether she's taken all her medication, feel concern about her eating and drinking, toss and turn in bed about getting her up for a doctor's appointment or feel anxious about what her mood will be like from moment to moment. I don't have to worry about balancing her crises or protecting her from accidents or realizing she had forgotten something and actually couldn't cope. I don't feel any better or worse for it.

Those piles of papers she had collected all around her and barricaded herself in with haven't yet shifted an inch. Sometimes I feel like I can release them and then sometimes I want to keep them close, as if one day I will finally be able to decipher their true import and meaning. I don't know whether I'll be able to let them go, in the same way that she didn't know either. They are significant as they represent her attempts to keep control in a life falling apart. Perhaps, riddled with grief as I am, I feel the need to hold to it all, her belongings, her letters and her little notes, to stop myself falling apart too. Just like Mum catalogued my life, I want to catalogue hers.

Mum was at the centre of so many threads, unconsciously woven into the fabric and tapestry of so many different lives. My mother's stories and memories are now my stories and memories, and they are very important to me. Her stories have become a part of who I am. I realize now that we all have the power to change other people's understanding of the world by sharing recollections and records of our own lived experiences. Our collective memories profoundly add to the richness of existence.

Understanding and uncovering the stories of the past is difficult, but they can be key to self-knowledge. I firmly believe that this is crucial to comprehending our present circumstances, ultimately directing us towards what our futures can hold.

Mum used to ask what I was scribbling as we chatted in her downstairs bedroom. She'd crinkle another toffee wrapper into the deep recesses of her cardigan pocket and say, **'What are you doing? Ay?** *Beta*? **What is so interesting, Shobi, about my life? I'm just an ordinary woman.'** I'd say, 'Your story is your story, Mum, and yours is an extraordinary life.'

A memory isn't simply a vision of the past. Memories can link people and places, and the loss of memory is more about the ways in which those links are slackened. With Mum, we discovered how to find new memory where links to the past were re-established and uncovered and remembered.

For it's not what you forget, it's what you remember.

P.S. 'Your daughter has had the royal stamp of approval. I've actually made it onto a British postage stamp, Mum.'

'Well that's nice, Shobi. Who would have thought the Queen would ever have noticed YOU? Did you go to the Post Office like that? Your hair, darling, looks like you've been dragged through a hedge backwards. Couldn't you just, for once, brush it nicely?'

I like to remember her like that.

Afterword from Alzheimer's Research UK

A diagnosis of dementia is a devastating blow. While for some it might make sense of confusing behaviours, actions out of type and personality changes, it nonetheless arrives with enormous uncertainty. When faced with a diagnosis of any condition, our immediate question is 'what can I expect?' With dementia, this is the hardest question to answer.

Fundamentally dementia is an incurable and progressive condition, and we know there will be no recovery. But how a dementia journey unfolds does not play to predictable patterns, and it makes the future for any person diagnosed, and their family, bleakly unknowable.

As Shobna Gulati outlines in *Remember Me*, each of us is unique, and each brain is unique, and as dementia unfolds, its impact will be idiosyncratic. Personality traits become exaggerated. Personality traits reverse. The usually sedate become irate, and robust characters wilt to wallflowers. The rules of our relationship with a person are torn up when dementia unfolds.

The symptoms themselves remain frequently underestimated. Many believe dementia to be a mild forgetfulness, an inconvenience of lost keys or forgotten names. The reality is more insidious as cognitive decline strips memory, ability and independence. And while memory loss characterizes many forms of dementia, it is profound in its nature. It is not forgetting where our keys might be, it is forgetting what they are for.

Memory loss to this degree cuts to the heart of identity. A great deal – perhaps all – of who we are emanates from memory. The present is the thinnest of veneers, and it is our formative experiences and their associated emotions, committed to memory, that create us as people. The loss, the reordering and the inconsistency of memory wreaked by dementia are acutely disorienting for the person and, of course, their carer.

This cognitive deterioration, and all its accompanying heartache, arrives as a result of damage to the brain. Another misconception of dementia – that it is just a by-product of age – overlooks this pathological reality. When someone is living with dementia, their brain is subject to atrophy – it shrinks – at many times the rate of normal aging. Cells in the brain are destroyed in multitudes and mass is lost. And with that our abilities, our memories and our connection to the world are lost too. A brain affected by Alzheimer's, the most common cause of dementia, can weigh about 140g less than a healthy brain. That's about the weight of an orange.

It's a startling image, but it is a reminder that we are dealing with physical disease processes, and this means research can give us hope. Scientists are discovering more about why cells are dying and how we might intervene to protect them. The coming years hold promise of new treatments that might act to slow the process down, rather than just papering over the cracks. We might soon welcome a day where treatment options offer hope of changing the lives of people with dementia – giving life back – in the same way we have achieved for those with cancer and heart disease.

While these efforts in the lab unfold, we need to remain focused on dementia education. The more we talk about our experiences, the more we normalize discourse around the condition and this is a hugely important step in truly taking it on.

A generation ago people talked in hushed tones about a loved one in the grip of a long illness. Then we started saying 'The Big C', and finally we began openly discussing our struggles with cancer. This has led to a huge public and government response to cancer and a research revolution. Now, over half of people live ten years or more beyond their diagnosis.

Perhaps we are now in 'The Big D' phase of dementia. We see and hear more stories of the reality of the condition than ever. There is increasing willingness to share our experiences, and Shobna Gulati's story – an honest, tender, funny, devastating depiction of how her mother was affected – is a continuation of this process. It will give confidence to others to do the same. Shobna's support of Alzheimer's Research UK in reaching South Asian communities in particular is a hugely important step towards normalizing discussion of dementia where stigma still prevails.

While for any individual or family dealing with dementia the future will feel uncertain and irrevocably changed, there is some help out there. Alzheimer's Research UK has a wealth of information about causes, symptoms, treatments and where to seek support. We will always make this freely available for those who need it on our website.

We can also help those affected and their carers to take part in research studies to help us better understand the condition and its impact in the brain. Where dementia can take so much away, participating in breakthrough research can return some agency to those affected. And it is research that will ultimately prevail in changing the story for millions living with dementia in the UK and around the world.

Tim Parry, Director, Alzheimer's Research UK
www.alzheimersresearchuk.org

Gratitude list

I am grateful.

This book came about because of a blog I was encouraged to write for Alzheimer's Research UK about my experience caring for my mum who had vascular dementia. It was posted on Twitter to help raise awareness and continue the conversation around the condition, highlighting specifically how dementia can sometimes be viewed by those from my background and heritage. The response was staggering: many came forward for the first time to share their powerful stories of joy and heartbreak with a desire to seek out information and support. So I'm starting with thanks to Laura Phipps, Lloyd Vaughan and Tim Parry from Alzheimer's Research UK, who have been incredibly supportive. The blog I wrote with Laura was spotted by the very talented Hamza Jahanzeb who brought it to the attention of the fantastically enthusiastic senior commissioning editor, Romilly Morgan (who took me into her heart) and the team at Octopus Books, where he worked at the time. I am incredibly grateful for their sincerity in backing me, for being behind a story which, though told from my perspective, also holds a universality. I couldn't have written this without the keen minds of Katherine Omerod and Charles Lauder, who have at times, in 'lockdown' when I have been struggling with my emotions and in the clutches of Covid-19, been able to brilliantly organize my thoughts without judgement or prejudice. To the wondrous wordsmith Lemn Sissay for giving this its first read, he has been an inspiration to me since I met him in Manchester in the late 1980s. He was there, right at the start, helping me to find the confidence to write, to find my voice by always putting me in front of a kind audience for my early poetry and stories. To the very patient and clever Pauline Bache, senior editor, who has painstakingly edited every step to page on lengthy Teams video calls in between cups of tea and scrambled eggs on oatcakes. To Peter for the gorgeous cover and all of the marketing and press team at Octopus Books, who have always listened and taken on my queries and reservations. To Victoria Young and Icon Books, for publishing my first essay on motherhood, in the collection of stories *Things I Wish I'd Known*.

To all my agents, 'Team Shobna' at Curtis Brown, who have been there for me on my creative journey over many years, to the terrific Lucy Morris from the literary team, who has looked after me through this and to Jonny Geller, who has always been there for me in my writing adventures.

To my uplifting friends and colleagues: Jayshri, Nitin, Bryan, Racheal, Nilam, Asye, Jag, Harold, Syreeta, Sangeeta, Dawinder, Kate, Armand, Lindsay, Paul, Jeanette, Tinge, Gini, Andrew, Musa, Tally, Keith, Joseph, Ali, Grant, Sam, Furquan, Tracey, Sandeep, Monica, Shaila, Rhys, David, Brasco, Nina, Richard, Miranda, Freda, Liz, Jill and Glen (Akshay's second mum and dad), Jonny C, Jonnie B, Gordon, Jamie, Abigail, Aulton, Nona, Uta, Rachel, Hannah, Sarah A, Janet, Becky, Anouska, Bex, Jo and all the fabulous 'Global Women' from our *Richard II* company, for their ongoing love and words of wisdom. Thanks all of you for listening, laughing, looking out for me and those who helped with starting my car, fixing things, making me delicious food, sending me vitamins and doing my shopping.

To Vic Wood.

To all my family.

To Søren, Nina and Rohan, who gave my sister, Sushma, unwavering support and blessing through all the challenging times.

To Aparna, Tarun and Aunty Chitra, who, on opposite sides of the world, have been on hand on WhatsApp, day and night, when my own command of Hindi/Punjabi has been dodgy (because it really is).

To my dear sister, Sushma, who has always said 'it's your story' and encouraged me, no matter how difficult it has been for all of us.

To my flamboyant, forward-thinking dad.

To my wonderful son, Akshay.

To my beautiful, graceful mum whose being and memories made this book.

THANK YOU.

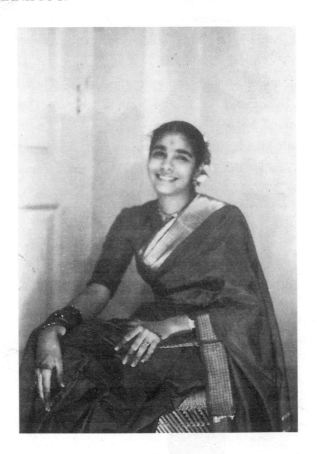